ωυ)Neued·O·

Coping Successfully with Hiatus Hernia

Dr Tom Smith has been a medical journalist and author since 1977, after spending six years in general practice and seven years in medical research. He continued in part-time practice until 2012. He has written regular columns in the *Scottish Sunday Mail*, *The Guardian*, the *Bradford Telegraph & Argus*, the *Carrick Gazette* and the *Galloway Gazette*. He still writes a weekly column for the *Lancashire Telegraph*. He has regular spots on BBC Radio Scotland in the *Morning Call* and *MacAulay and Co.* programmes. He has written three humorous books on his experiences in practice: *A Seaside Practice*, *Going Loco* and *Doctor, Have You Got A Minute?*, all published by Short Books. His other books for Sheldon Press include *Physical Intelligence*, *Heart Attacks: Prevent and Survive*, *Living with Alzheimer's Disease*, *Coping Successfully with Prostate Cancer*, *Overcoming Back Pain*, *Coping with Bowel Cancer*, *Coping with Heartburn and Reflux*, *Coping with Age-related Memory Loss*, *Skin Cancer: Prevent and Survive*, *How to Get the Best from Your Doctor*, *Coping with Kidney Disease* and *Osteoporosis: Prevent and Treat*.

Overcoming Common Problems Series

Selected titles

A full list of titles is available from Sheldon Press,
36 Causton Street, London SW1P 4ST and on our website at
www.sheldonpress.co.uk

Overcoming Common Problems

Coping Successfully with Hiatus Hernia

Second edition

DR TOM SMITH

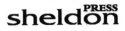

*This book is for all the people at Sheldon
who have helped me over the years*

First published in Great Britain in 1997

Sheldon Press
36 Causton Street
London SW1P 4ST
www.sheldonpress.co.uk

Reprinted four times
Reissued 2011
Reprinted once
Second edition published 2014

British Library Cataloguing-in-Publication Data
A catalogue record for this book is available from the British Library

ISBN 978–1–84709–339–4
eBook ISBN 978–1–84709–340–0

Typeset by Fakenham Prepress Solutions, Fakenham, Norfolk NR21 8NN
First printed in Great Britain by Ashford Colour Press
Subsequently digitally reprinted in Great Britain

eBook by Fakenham Prepress Solutions, Fakenham, Norfolk NR21 8NN

Produced on paper from sustainable forests

Contents

Note to the reader

This is not a medical book and is not intended to replace advice from your doctor. Consult your pharmacist or doctor if you believe you have any of the symptoms described, and if you think you might need medical help.

Introduction

People with 'indigestion', 'dyspepsia', 'heartburn' and 'stomach upsets' have been buying patent medicine pills and potions in their millions for over a hundred years. They buy them again and again, so that the medication becomes a normal part of everyday routine – as if it is normal, rather than unusual, to have such symptoms.

They often assume that the cause of their symptoms is a sensitive stomach, or an allergy or even a stomach ulcer. They may even blame the food, so that they avoid fries, or any food which they ate immediately before the symptoms arose. It is so easy to assume that a particular food has a special effect on the stomach, when in fact there is strong evidence that the stomach is a very tolerant organ. A normal stomach allows us to widen enormously the range of foods we can eat without a moment's complaint or thought.

So why do so many people take indigestion remedies so often? For some there may be an element of gastritis – inflammation of the stomach. A few will have an ulcer. But for many more of us the true cause is a hiatus hernia.

This book is about hiatus hernias. It explains simply what they are, why they cause symptoms, how the symptoms can be relieved, and how people with hiatus hernias can live a normal life – without having constant problems. A hiatus hernia is not a complicated condition, and if it is kept under control, it can be so easy to live with that it can almost be forgotten. But it does demand attention to lifestyle, as well as to its medical management and treatment. And for some people it may mean surgery.

Coping Successfully with Hiatus Hernia covers all aspects of the care of people with a hiatus hernia. It is meant for sufferers and for their partners and carers. It is based on the principle that if you, as a patient, know why you are asked to do (or not do) something, you will find it easier to comply with the advice. You will learn why it is better not to take the risk of bending over, or lying flat, and when new symptoms should force you to see your doctor, rather than treat yourself. It will also guide you on when your symptoms are *not* likely to be due to your hernia, but may be caused by something else. Hiatus hernia often causes chest-pain, but so do heart and lung problems, and there may be a time when you need to know the difference – which is why I have devoted a chapter to sorting them out.

However, this is not a book to cause concern or worry – in fact it is just the reverse. Its tone is upbeat, positively optimistic – because there are many ways in which the symptoms of a hiatus hernia can be minimized and its complications prevented, and most of them are under your own control. Hiatus hernia is a condition whose outcome, for the vast majority of people, depends almost entirely on themselves.

Of course, medical, and sometimes surgical, treatment does help, and for a few it is crucial. But if you can face up to the demands (in most cases they are the pleasures) of a new lifestyle, you will almost certainly relieve your own symptoms and avoid the need for specialist or hospital care.

Hiatus hernia can affect all ages and both sexes, so this book is for everyone who has been diagnosed as having a hiatus hernia, or who thinks that they may have one. You may recognize yourself among the case histories in Chapter 1. If so, please read on.

1

A few fellow-sufferers

In this chapter are a few case histories of hiatus hernia sufferers. They are all typical of the people who suffer from the complaint, though their symptoms differ widely. So if you don't relate to the first story, read on – you will probably see yourself in one of the others. And don't worry if you don't immediately understand all the details of the stories, or the terms used – you'll find them explained in later chapters, and in the Glossary at the end of the book.

Mary's story

Mary was 58 when she first visited her doctor. Since her children had left home (she had been a full-time home-maker), and her life had become less hectic, she had put on a few stones in weight, so that she had what is politely called a matronly figure. To put it more bluntly, she was about five feet three tall (1.6 m) and weighed more than 12 stones (75 kg).

Her 'indigestion' symptoms had started about four years before. At first, she'd felt a sharp, raw pain in the centre of her chest, with an occasional sour taste in the mouth, that came on shortly after meals (or even a cup of tea), particularly when she was putting her feet up. She noticed, too, that the symptoms came on when she bent down, either to get things from low-down in the kitchen, or when she was weeding the garden.

She assumed that this was to do with her increased weight or her age, or even the fact that she had started to wear a support girdle – so she decided not to bother her doctor, and to treat herself. She started taking indigestion pills – antacids such as Rennies – and, to begin with, thought no more of her symptoms.

For the first few months, the antacids always eased her symptoms. In fact, they did so very quickly, far faster than she might have expected if the problem were inside her stomach – and that might have given her a clue that the problem was further up, in her oesophagus (the tube leading from her throat to the stomach).

However, this honeymoon period did not last. Gradually she found herself taking antacids every day. The pain lasted longer, came on more often, and was spreading further up into her chest. To ease it she started to drink copious amounts of milk and to eat biscuits, which did nothing for her weight problem. The character of her pain, too, had changed. It was by now clearly recognizable as heartburn – a burning sensation which she felt in a vertical line down the middle of her chest.

Even that was not enough to take her to the doctor. She assumed that heartburn was a common complaint, which could be dealt with by over-the-counter medicines, and not the sort of problem with which to bother her doctor. So she carried on self treating with antacids, and lashings of milk and biscuits.

Two further developments finally brought her to her senses – and to the doctor's surgery. The first was a persistent, dull ache right in the centre of her chest, just behind the inverted V at the lower end of her breastbone. It never seemed to go away completely, and sometimes woke her at night. The second was less regular but just as worrying. The sour taste in the mouth had not only become much more frequent, but was worse, in that she found her mouth filling with sour, watery material that had apparently welled up from her stomach (a substance known as waterbrash). This was sometimes so bad that it made her choke. Along with this, she found that she could no longer lie flat in bed at night, particularly if she lay on her right side. This invariably produced the waterbrash, and occasionally her mouth filled with the food that she had eaten an hour or so before. This happened one night in her sleep, and she awoke terrified – literally drowning on a mouthful of semi-digested milk.

The next morning, in something approaching a panic, she saw her doctor, who had no difficulty making the diagnosis of a sliding hiatus hernia (see Chapter 3), but who would have preferred knowing about it at a much earlier stage! Then her treatment would have been easier, and there would have been much less damage to reverse.

Eve's story

Eve was 40 when she noticed her first symptoms. Married with teenage children, Eve was an only daughter and had recently had to take into her home her father, who was in the later stages of Alzheimer's disease. A worrier at the best of times, Eve's stress then was huge, and she was in no doubt that this was a direct cause of her symptoms.

However, her hernia did not show itself in pain or waterbrash. Instead, she had what she described as discomfort – a feeling that the food she had swallowed had not gone all the way into her stomach, but had stuck somewhere in the middle of her chest. This prevented her from eating any more, so that meals were a real trial for her. There were times when she could not eat any solid food – indeed, was frightened of doing so, in case it stuck. So she tended to stick to semi-solid foods and liquids, feeling that they would go down more easily. As they tended to be minced meats and milky puddings, she started to put on weight.

Quite the opposite of Mary's case, however, she found that lying down actually helped her symptoms. Resting, when she could grab a minute, always seemed to allow something inside her to relax and let the food slide into the stomach. Her symptoms never started when she was in bed, and she never had a burning sensation or the flow of water-brash into her mouth.

Her doctor at the time, worried about the symptoms of food sticking in her chest, arranged for a barium-swallow X-ray examination, which showed a small hiatus hernia. This surprised him, as he was looking for other conditions more likely to produce these symptoms of blockage – the main one in women of Eve's age being achalasia, in which the lower end of the oesophagus goes into spasm (a form of cramp), which eases with rest. But the barium showed quite clearly a rolling hiatus hernia, and he was happy to advise her on that basis. (Achalasia and the different types of hiatus hernia will be explained in more detail in Chapter 3, along with the other conditions with which hiatus hernia can be confused.)

After her father died, and the main source of stress had gone, her symptoms stopped. For 20 years, they did not return. Last year, Eve – now 60 years old, and a healthy woman – developed a severe attack of shingles. Unfortunately, she first noticed the rash, which ran around the right side of her chest over her breast, only at midday on a Saturday. Being considerate, she did not want to disturb her doctor at the weekend, so she treated herself until the Monday morning – with calamine lotion.

This was a mistake – it is vital that shingles are treated within the first 36 hours (preferably 24 hours) with the antiviral drug acyclovir (Zovirax). Acyclovir damps down the eruption, greatly eases the pain and, most important, helps you avoid the sometimes very severe post-shingles pain in the scarred area of skin left by the acute attack.

By Monday, Eve's shingles were a mess. There was a thick band of pustules and inflamed skin from the spine to her breastbone on the right side of her chest, and she was in severe pain and considerable distress. At this point, her hiatus hernia symptoms returned. Once again, eating produced this feeling of blockage. She had to confine her eating to porridge, soup and custard, as nothing solid would go down. No amount of swallowing, she felt, would 'push the food down'. One crucial symptom was the pressing desire to belch. She had the ever present feeling that there was gas in her chest or upper stomach, and that she would get relief if only she could bring it up. But she found it impossible to do so. She thought that liquid antacids might help, and scoured the pharmacy for the best – but none helped her. Changing her body position did not help either. She spent hours rolling around in her chair or bed trying to find a position to give her relief from the gas or the 'blockage', but it was all in vain.

Her doctor was convinced that the painkillers, which she was taking for the shingles, had stimulated the return of the hernia symptoms. He therefore prescribed a drug to reduce any irritation in the stomach, while continuing with the painkillers. She gradually recovered from both the pain and the hernia symptoms, but it took her more than four months to feel confident enough to eat solid foods again. Six months after the onset of the shingles attack, she is back to her normal self.

She still tends to avoid lumpy foods (she makes sure she chews everything thoroughly before swallowing), and has got into the habit of eating several small meals a day, rather than three larger meals, because she feels uncomfortable with a full stomach. She avoids bending down – but only because she has heard that it is not good for a hiatus hernia, not because bending has ever bothered her! She no longer takes any medication, and is doing well.

Harry's story

Harry is 68 and a retired electrician. His symptoms started when he was in his early fifties – with hiccups! They would come on late at night, in bed, just before he dropped off to sleep. He noticed that they were more likely to start if he'd had sweets, cream or chocolate just before going to bed (he admitted to a very sweet tooth). At the same time he felt what he described as discomfort (it wasn't painful or burning) in the upper middle region of his stomach, and a bloated feeling deep in his chest, as if gases were trapped inside it. Like Eve, at times like this he desperately wanted to belch, but couldn't. He assumed that this was just a reaction to eating too many sweet things, and changed his late evening habits. He took a glass of warm milk instead, which helped a little. Even then, the hiccups sometimes occurred when he lay down flat in bed. The only way to relieve them was to get up and walk around, or sit up and read. Putting extra pillows on his side of the bed helped, too. Being propped up at an angle of around 45 degrees kept the symptoms at bay, and seemed to prevent the hiccups. After a few restless nights he became more used to sleeping in that position.

Ten years ago, things changed. While at work one day, crawling around under the floorboards of a house he was rewiring, Harry developed a severe pain in the centre of his chest, felt very sick, and broke out into a cold, clammy sweat. A doctor was called, and Harry was admitted to hospital with a suspected heart attack.

However, the hospital tests showed that these new symptoms were actually caused by an inflamed gall-bladder, which was full of gallstones. It was assumed that his other symptoms were also related to his gall-bladder disease, so that when the gall-bladder was removed a few weeks later, Harry expected his hiccups and discomfort to disappear. They didn't.

While the surgeons were removing his gall-bladder, they checked on his diaphragm, and confirmed that he had a hiatus hernia. However, they considered it not to be serious enough for a surgical repair, and left it as it was.

Since then, Harry has been careful. He has had no recurrence of his gall-bladder symptoms, though occasionally has his evening hiccups and discomfort – but if he avoids bending over and eating anything after around 8 p.m., he remains relatively symptom-free. Recently he has been having the odd bout of heartburn, for which he takes one tablet of ranitidine (Zantac) a day, and that seems to help.

Two other changes in his life may also have contributed to his improvement: the first is that now he has retired he no longer has to crawl around in confined spaces or lie on a floor with head and chest down a hole, working with electrical wiring. That must be about the worst occupation for anyone with a hiatus hernia! The other is that he has stopped smoking. He is living proof that someone can stop smoking after 40 years, and feel much the better for it. It will certainly have done his stomach and hiatus hernia a power of good, as well, of course, as his lungs, heart and blood vessels.

And now that he has retired, he has taken up golf. That keeps him fit, and with the exercise he has shed about two stones (13 kg) in weight. This, too, may well have improved the state of his hernia. He did think of taking up bowls, but was strongly advised against it – bowls is no game for anyone with a hiatus hernia.

Harry does illustrate an important point. One in every five people with hiatus hernia has another related illness. The list includes duodenal and gastric ulcers, gallstones, and coronary heart disease, so that even if a hiatus hernia has been proved by an X-ray (as in Eve's and Mary's cases), or by its being seen during surgery (as in Harry's case), it should never be assumed that any symptoms around the upper stomach and chest are due to the hernia. That pain in the chest could be angina or a heart attack, and a pain in the upper stomach could be due to an ulcer or gallstones. So if new symptoms arise, and they don't go away with the usual treatment, or are worse than usual, don't hesitate to seek urgent advice. It can often be difficult to distinguish between the pain of hiatus hernia and of heart attack, but one thing is sure – taking an antacid usually eases hiatus hernia pain very quickly. It will make not a jot of difference to heart pain.

James's story

James, at 50, was a fairly stubborn man. A schoolteacher, he had no use for doctors, and felt that he could look after himself very well without them. That may have been true when he was younger, but he had a failing that was nearly the death of him. He enjoyed his 'little drink' in the evenings. That varied from a scalding hot cup of tea to a neat whisky, neither of which was compatible with his hiatus hernia, which he had treated himself for many years.

He had started to have mild heartburn when he was in his late thirties. It was worse just after a meal – which for James, who lived on his own, was usually a fry-up – so he always kept a bottle of his favourite antacid mixture beside the kitchen sink. A day never passed without a swig from his white bottle.

As the years passed, however, the symptoms worsened. With every meal, he experienced a deep-seated pain behind the lower half of his breastbone, in the centre of his chest. It was at its worst if the food was hot or if he drank alcohol with it or after it. Hot tea, a neat whisky or even a white wine brought it on. At the same time, his heartburn was more severe than before, and lasted longer. He was getting through more white bottles every week, and was also taking anti-indigestion tablets by the dozen per week.

This deterioration was gradual, so that even his new intensity of pain did not cause him to seek his doctor's advice. He had to be shocked into doing that. When he got out of bed one morning, he felt dizzy and faint. He staggered to the toilet, where he passed a motion that was the colour and consistency of warm tar. He looked pale, and felt cold and clammy. He knew this could not be right, and called the emergency number.

It was lucky that he did, because the black stool was a sign of bleeding – and the bleeding had come from an ulcer in his oesophagus. Over the years, his oesophagus had become chronically inflamed from the back-flow of acid from his stomach, and this had eventually eroded into a blood-vessel. James had been on the edge of a precipice for many months, and was in immediate danger of dying from a massive internal haemorrhage.

His story has a happy ending. James was rushed to hospital, where intensive medical treatment saved his life. He is now under constant medical supervision, and is being persuaded to change his lifestyle – mainly his eating and drinking habits – by a new partner, who is a much better cook than he is!

James's hernia was complicated by the fact that he also had a Barrett's oesophagus, a condition in which the lowest region of the oesophagus is much more prone than normal to ulceration. This will be explained in more detail in Chapter 3. Suffice it to say here that the combination of Barrett's oesophagus and hiatus hernia can at times be life-threatening – besides causing bleeding, it can also perforate, so that the stomach contents can be expelled into the chest cavity, where they cause a very severe, acute illness. James could have paid for his relative self-neglect with his life.

Jane's story

Bleeding from oesophagitis (inflammation of the oesophagus) need not be as dramatic as in James's case, but it can, in the long term, be just as severe. Jane, at 62, had known she had a hiatus hernia for years, but was happy that she had it under good control. About five years before, she'd had what she called 'a flare-up', with the typical heartburn, water-brash and swallowing problems described in Mary's case. However, it had settled down with medical treatment, and she had gradually drifted away from her doctor's care, deciding to buy her antacids and ranitidine from the pharmacy and to do her own thing, rather than spend time waiting in the practice queue for her repeat prescriptions. She was a busy woman, and with a small florist's shop to manage she had other things to do with her time.

She still had the odd bout of heartburn, but tended to ignore it until just before Christmas last year, when she had a ten-fold increase in her workload. Being the best and most reliable florist in her small town, she was in great demand for Christmas floral decorations and wreaths. Being a very conscientious (some might say obsessional) woman, she did all the work herself. Last year, for the first time ever, she couldn't fulfil her contracts. She had to hire another woman to complete them because she was just too exhausted to carry on. After standing for an hour or so, she was dizzy, faint, and gasping for breath. She looked pale and drawn, and could feel her heart racing and thumping.

Accepting at last that there was something seriously wrong, she dragged herself along to her doctor. He took one look at her and tested her haemoglobin level – a measurement of her red blood cells. It was less than half of what it should have been.

Jane's case is quite common. Sometimes self-treatment serves only to mask the symptoms, leaving the lower end of the oesophagus still irritated by the stomach's digestive juices (as explained in Chapter 3). That can lead to the loss of tiny amounts of blood, every day, into the digestive system. It may be so small that it does not show obviously in the stool, but over the years the blood-loss adds up. It is impossible for the bone marrow, which makes new red blood-cells, to keep up with the extra demand, and the person becomes very anaemic. That may not show itself in symptoms – until there is a need to step up a gear physically. Then the need for extra oxygen can't be met unless the remaining red blood-cells are asked to do at least double their usual work – which means pumping them twice as fast round the body. This forces the heart to work much harder than normal. It can be the last straw, and the result is exhaustion.

So the ramifications of a hiatus hernia extend much further than just the symptoms arising from an irritation at the lower end of the oesophagus. That is why, if you have a hiatus hernia, your doctor will, once in a while, check on your haemoglobin level, to see if you are becoming anaemic. It is simply a matter of a small blood sample, either from a finger-tip or a vein, once every three months or so.

Billy's story

Occasionally a hiatus hernia arises in people in whom you least expect it. Billy, aged 25, was a fitness fanatic. He trained at his local gym five days a week. He ran, had a special routine on all the machines, and finished by lifting weights. He knew enough not to get muscle-bound, and to take two days a week off to let his muscles relax and build up the stores of energy that had been used by the exercise.

So he was a super-fit man in peak condition. Yet he appeared in his doctor's consulting room complaining of a pain behind his breastbone and acid regurgitation into his mouth when he bent over or lifted weights. He also found he couldn't breathe as deeply as he used to, and was even getting breathless with exercise, an unheard of problem for him. He'd had these symptoms for about a month, and they were not getting easier.

It was only with more detailed questioning that he admitted that the symptoms followed a particular incident in the gym, about which he had been a bit embarrassed. He had been fooling about with friends, he said. They were comparing the strength of their stomach muscles – which in his case was pretty impressive! The challenge was to take a blow in the stomach with a medicine ball, thrown as hard as possible at close range. The first few shots were no bother to him, because he was ready for them, and kept his muscles tense. But a friend had caught him unawares, with stomach wall relaxed, and the ball had hit him full in the upper abdomen.

It had hurt a lot, but his macho pride kept him from admitting it, and he had rested for the next two or three days to let the pain subside. The hiatus hernia symptoms had started a few days later. This is a familiar story: a sharp blow in the abdomen with a blunt object may leave no external scars or bruises, but can rupture organs inside. Harry Houdini, the great escapologist, used to challenge people to punch him in the stomach as hard as they liked: he was always able to receive the punch with equanimity because he tensed his muscles beforehand. The one time someone punched him unexpectedly, he died from a ruptured appendix.

The same might have happened to Billy. Instead, he sustained a small rupture in his diaphragm, around the opening through which the oesophagus ran. A plain X-ray (no barium was needed) showed that quite a lot of his stomach had slipped up into his chest. He needed surgery to put it back into the abdomen and repair the hole in his diaphragm. He was lucky: if his bowel had given way instead, he would have been desperately ill.

His was an unusual way to start off a hiatus hernia, but it is by no means an isolated case. Many people suffer the effects of being hit in the stomach with blunt instruments: it happens in road accidents, in falls at work, in the home and at play. People have sustained ruptured diaphragms falling off horses and off mountains, or off ladders when doing DIY at home or pruning fruit trees. Often they have other, more obvious injuries, which occupy the casualty team's time, and the possibility of a diaphragm tear is missed. So if your symptoms of hiatus hernia have arisen out of the blue, try to think of any possible incident which might have caused it. It may just be a pointer for your doctor to follow in his study of your case.

This book would not be complete without mention of two special categories of hiatus hernia – in pregnancy and in babies. The following two case histories describe them.

Liz's story

Liz, at 23, was sailing blissfully through a very successful and happy first pregnancy when she ran up against her first symptoms of hiatus hernia. It started in the sixth month, with heartburn and acid regurgitation into the mouth, especially when she was lying down. She also found she could only take small amounts of food at a time without feeling full. At night, the heartburn kept her from settling, and even when she did drop off to sleep, she was soon wakened by it.

The reason for her symptoms was that the baby was filling her abdomen, and pushing her stomach up into her chest. That didn't help her breathing either, so she became very easily breathless.

Happily there was good news for her on two counts. First, pregnancy hiatus hernia is usually reversed as soon as the baby is born. In fact, it eases a lot in the last month, when the baby's head settles into the pelvis, and leaves a little more room for the stomach to return to its normal anatomical position. Secondly, the hiatus hernia is relatively easily treated even while you are still pregnant. Remaining upright (even sleeping upright) is a great help, and there are several proprietary and prescription medicines which ease the heartburn very quickly and reliably. Liz was given the appropriate advice and medicines, and the heartburn vanished, as promised, after the birth. She has not had it since. She was reassured that the pregnancy did no permanent damage to her diaphragm, oesophagus or stomach.

Martha's story

Martha had reached the age of 78 with no serious illness of note. She prided herself that she had 'kept out of her doctor's way for more than three-quarters of a century' (with the exception of her pregnancies, of course). Then she started to have difficulties in swallowing, so that she could only drink a little without feeling that 'something was sticking'. Added to that, she was continually belching, which was most embarrassing. She was also losing weight rapidly. Yet she tolerated these symptoms for three weeks before they forced her finally to see her doctor. By this time she was constantly feeling sick and was retching, but could not actually vomit, though she desperately wanted to.

Clearly something serious had happened suddenly – but what could it be? She had no fever, though she was dehydrated and had a pulse rate of more than 100 beats per minute. Her doctor could find nothing wrong with her heart or her breathing. Admitted to hospital, a chest X-ray and a CT scan of her chest and abdomen identified the problem. She was rehydrated with plenty of intravenous fluids and prepared for surgery that day.

Her GP had thought of several possible diagnoses before sending her to hospital, such as an oesophageal obstruction due to cancer or to a stricture from oesophagitis, or even a problem with the ability of the muscles in the oesophagus to manage the forward passage of food into the stomach (a 'motility disorder' such as achalasia – see p. 34). None of these diagnoses really fitted with the sudden onset of Martha's symptoms and her distress at being unable to be sick.

The X-rays and scans revealed the answer. She had had a paraoesophageal hernia for many years – without it causing her any significant discomfort or symptoms that would lead her to seek advice. Eventually, however, at the junction with her oesophagus, her stomach had twisted around through more than a right angle, and this had blocked off any chance of food passing downwards through the twisted area, and of course had prevented any of the stomach contents from passing upwards. She could neither swallow nor vomit, despite her desperately wishing to do both.

This condition is called gastric volvulus, and is usually restricted to older people, but it is one that doctors always need to keep in mind when dealing with what might be mistaken for, say, a severe gastroenteritis. Any delay in correcting the twisted stomach can lead to its blood supply being compromised, which of course could well be rapidly fatal.

Happily, the surgeons were able to use laparoscopic surgery (see p. 87) to untwist the stomach, fix it securely to the back wall of her abdomen, and repair her (very long-standing) hiatus hernia. She was able to go home within four days of her admission feeling better than she had done, she admitted finally, for years.

Peter's story

Peter is three years old now, and a very lively and lovable little terror. It is difficult to reconcile this with the fact that he spent most of his first year strapped into a special chair to keep him upright, day and night. It took courage and patience in large measure from both parents to help him through that year.

Peter's mother first became concerned when, at about six weeks old, he started to vomit back his feeds after being laid down to rest in the cot. It happened so often that she began to worry that there was some form of obstruction in the bowel. This fear was reinforced by her finding that he was no longer putting on the expected weight for a healthy baby. She spoke about her fears to her health visitor, who arranged a 'test feed' with her doctor.

One possible diagnosis for a six-week-old baby boy who is vomiting is pyloric stenosis – a benign overgrowth of muscle-tissue around the outlet of the stomach into the duodenum, which blocks the flow of blood from the stomach to the rest of the bowel. During a test feed, the doctor can feel the overgrowth – it feels like a hazel-nut – in the upper abdomen. A child with pyloric stenosis shoots the vomit out, like a bullet from a gun (it is called projectile vomiting) – and this occurs regardless of the child's posture.

However, Peter's story did not sound right for pyloric stenosis. His vomit just flowed out of his mouth, but only when he was horizontal. In Peter's case the presence of a hiatus hernia was suggested by small flecks of blood in the vomit, showing that there was already some degree of oesophageal irritation from the stomach contents (described further in Chapter 3).

A barium X-ray (they can be done on a six-week-old) confirmed the hernia. The next decision was what to do about it. Most early hernias like this will settle on their own if left to do so – and the way to do it was to keep Peter upright for the rest of the first year of his life! That may seem cruel, but he took to the regime beautifully. He stopped vomiting, put on plenty of weight, and developed into a healthy, normal child. Now, at three years old, he is a very lively toddler.

It is important to diagnose a congenital hiatus hernia like this early on, because if it is missed or left for many months, the lower end of the oesophagus can become scarred, and may leave the child with a short oesophagus. This leaves the junction between the oesophagus and the stomach higher up than it should be – in the chest cavity rather than below the diaphragm – which may require extensive surgery later.

These aren't the only symptoms of a hiatus hernia in children. It may show itself for the first time in an older child, say around a year old, as peculiar writhing movements of the neck. The mother often interprets them as some sort of fit, which naturally causes great concern and anxiety. It is only when the contortions are related to swallowing that the reason for them becomes clear. The child is using these movements in an attempt to get the food that is sticking in the oesophagus down into the stomach. Children are quite conscious of what they are doing, but are obviously not old enough to explain why.

Once the diagnosis of hiatus hernia has been made in a child, and the treatment has been successful (this is described in Chapter 5), it is still important to follow up its progress for many years – at least into adulthood. For about half of all children who are treated for it go on to have the adult-type hiatus hernia – and this has to be treated properly. This, too, is discussed in more detail in Chapter 5.

Reading back through all these cases it becomes clear that hiatus hernia is not just a single condition. It has many forms, and produces different sets of symptoms in different people. To understand why this should be, you need to know something about the normal oesophagus, diaphragm and stomach, and how the normal anatomy and architecture can go wrong. This information is given in Chapter 2.

2

The normal oesophagus, diaphragm and stomach

The swallowing mechanism

Before learning about hiatus hernia you must know something about the normal workings of the oesophagus, the diaphragm and the stomach (see Figure 1). The first thing to understand is the action of normal swallowing. The only part of swallowing of which we are normally conscious happens at the back of our tongue and in our throat. From then on, after the food or drink reaches the top of the oesophagus, the process is an active but unconscious one in the oesophagus. It is completed when the food enters the stomach.

It is easy to imagine that the oesophagus is an inactive tube, through which the material we have swallowed passes, by gravity, to the stomach. What really happens in swallowing is very different. We transfer food towards the back of our throat (the pharynx) using our tongue. Once the food reaches the pharynx, swallowing becomes automatic: that is, we can feel the food in our throat, but we cannot stop the action of swallowing. This is now under the control of our autonomic nervous system, which also controls the movement of our food through the rest of the gut, without our being aware of it.

We divide the autonomic (also called subconscious or involuntary) phase of swallowing into two: what goes on in the pharynx and what happens in the oesophagus.

In the pharynx

When food or drink hits the pharynx (the back of the throat), it stimulates two muscle reflexes: one shuts off the passages back into the mouth, the back of the nose, and the lungs; the other squeezes the food down into the top of the oesophagus. The aim of this is to

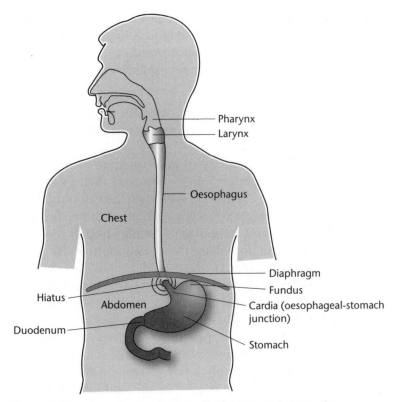

Figure 1 The normal oesophagus, diaphragm and stomach

ensure that we do not inhale and swallow at the same time – food in the lungs is a disaster that can lead to very sudden death.

In the oesophagus

The oesophagus is a very muscular tube: the action of the autonomic nerves causes it to contract and relax in a very co-ordinated fashion, so that it actively pushes solids and liquids onwards into the stomach. These rippling muscle contractions, called peristalsis, occur through the whole length of the gut, from oesophagus to anus, and are the means by which food, and then faeces, are passed onwards. If that process fails, the food just sticks: any liquid may trickle downwards, but solids will stay in a lump, stretching the tube walls, and causing considerable discomfort.

There are three recognizable types of muscle contraction in the oesophagus.

1 Once we start to swallow, primary peristaltic waves ripple down the oesophagus, pushing food in front of them, at a rate of five centimetres per second.

2 If the primary peristaltic waves don't manage to empty the contents of the oesophagus into the stomach, then a secondary peristaltic wave starts, about half way down the oesophagus.This reinforces the primary wave, and sometimes it can be felt as an uncomfortable, almost indescribable feeling, deep in the chest. This may have been, for example, the reason for the discomfort in Eve's case (see Chapter 1).

3 Tertiary muscle contractions in the oesophagus have been iden- tified by radiologists, with their vast experience of watching barium-swallow X-rays. These occur in one segment of oesopha- gus at a time: they don't appear to be involved in swallowing, and don't propel food onwards. Their purpose is unknown: it is possible that they are simply a way of keeping the muscles in tone between meals, while waiting for the next lump of food to come down!

Peristalsis – both primary and secondary – is vital for transfer- ring solid and semi-solid food from the back of the pharynx into the stomach. As long as we are upright when we drink, however, peristalsis isn't absolutely necessary for liquids. Once we have swal- lowed a liquid, as long as there is no obstruction to its flow, it will reach the stomach by gravity alone. However, peristalsis is needed to ensure that food cannot return to the throat. Without it, if you swallowed when lying flat, or even standing upside down, the food or drink would flow back into your mouth.

I have very graphic memories of being taught, at medical school, about the way the oesophagus works. Our physiology lecturer, Dr Hilary Harries, brought into the lecture hall a pint of beer, climbed on to the demonstration table, stood on his head, facing us, then drank the beer in one go, upside down. He had no difficulty doing so, and he did not spill a drop. He declined to perform an encore!

So the rippling muscles in the wall of the oesophagus ensure that passage of food and drink is one-way only. This is very important: if food travels in the opposite direction, not only are you sick, but you feel terrible with it.

At its lower end, the oesophagus passes through a hole – the hiatus – in the diaphragm, a sheet of muscle which separates the contents of the chest from those of the abdomen (the diaphragm is described more fully later in the chapter). Below the diaphragmatic hiatus, the oesophagus becomes the upper part of the stomach. How it does so, and how it relates to the diaphragm, are crucial in determining whether or not you have a hiatus hernia.

The junction of oesophagus and stomach

If it is important that food flows in a one-way direction within the oesophagus, it is even more vital that, once it has reached the stomach, it stays there, and can only travel onwards into the duodenum. The digestive juices inside the stomach are very acidic, and designed to digest proteins. The stomach-wall is extremely well protected against its own juices with a thick layer of mucus (to protect against the protein-digesting enzymes) and bicarbonate (to protect against the acid). However, the oesophagus is not at all protected in this way – gastric juices which get into the oesophagus are a powerful irritant. They can cause ulcers, inflammation, friability and eventually scarring at the lower end of the oesophagus (as discussed in Chapter 3).

There are therefore several mutually co-operative mechanisms which act to ensure that, once food has entered the stomach, it can't flow backwards, up into the oesophagus.

The cardia

The last five centimetres or so of the oesophagus lie under the diaphragm within the abdominal cavity (see Figure 1). The oesophagus meets the stomach at its upper right-hand surface, not quite at the top – if the stomach were a clock-face, and you were looking at it from the front, then the junction between the oesophagus and the stomach is at about 11 o'clock.

This junction is called the cardia. It meets the stomach at an angle so that the food slides easily into the bottom 90 per cent of the stomach. This process is not unlike tipping a glass to one side when you pour your drink into it, to avoid turbulence and froth. The angle should also ensure that, if there is any reverse movement of food upwards within the stomach, it passes by the entry from the oesophagus and ends up in the top part of the stomach – continuing the analogy with a clock face, the 12 o'clock area. This is called the fundus.

The fundus, being the uppermost part of the stomach, which is virtually like an unexpanded balloon, is a safety valve which gathers any gas that has been swallowed or produced in the process of digestion. It sits neatly under the diaphragm.

The sphincter

At the cardia, just where the oesophagus becomes the stomach, there is a ring of muscle around it, within its wall. Imagine it is an elastic band around the tube, gripping it a little and narrowing it. This is called the gastro-oesophageal sphincter. There are sphincters at several crucial sites in the gut: besides the one between oesophagus and stomach, they also occur at the outlet of the stomach into the duodenum, between the small bowel and large bowel, and at the anus. They control the passage of food and food residues from one segment of the digestive system to the next, and prevent back-flow.

So not only is the angle at which the oesophagus meets the stomach important, so is the efficiency of the gastro-oesophageal sphincter. It opens (i.e. the ring of muscle relaxes) to let food and drink pass from oesophagus to stomach, and it closes (the ring of muscle contracts) to prevent the digesting food flowing back from stomach to oesophagus. In effect, it is a one-way valve.

As well as the sphincter muscles, there is another system of muscles that keeps this valve-structure intact. These are the oblique muscle-fibres in the wall of the oesophagus and stomach around the sphincter, which keep oesophagus and stomach at the appropriate angle to each other, in a sling-like support. Without them the angle between oesophagus and stomach would flatten out, and the bottom end of the oesophagus would be more open to back-flow pressures.

Such back-flow pressures are normal when the stomach, full of food, starts its job of digestion. Like the oesophagus, the stomach wall is subject to peristalsis, and although the movement is usually from above down, there are also chaotic churning waves, designed to mix the stomach contents thoroughly with the digestive juices. If the sphincter and the oblique muscle-fibres are not working properly, then this may push the stomach contents into the lower end of the oesophagus – with the irritant consequences described above.

Abdominal pressure

An essential force to prevent that back-flow is the positive pressure in the abdominal cavity. The biggest difference between the chest and abdominal cavities is the pressure within them: inside the chest, the pressure must be kept relatively low, or the lungs could not expand; inside the abdomen, the pressure is much higher, because external pressure on the gut helps to push its contents onwards and eventually, of course, out. The organ that maintains this big differential in pressure between the abdominal and chest cavities is the diaphragm.

The diaphragm

The diaphragm is a tough sheet of muscle which is attached in an umbrella-shaped circle around the lower margin of the ribs. Above it are the lungs and the heart; below it are the kidneys (to left and right), the liver (on the right side), the spleen (on the left side) and all the gut from the stomach through the small and large bowel, to the rectum and anus. The high pressure within the abdomen means that if the muscles of the diaphragm aren't working properly (either because of an inherited fault, or because they have given way under pressure), some part of the contents of the abdomen can be pushed into the chest cavity. This is what is meant by a hernia.

Obviously the diaphragm is not a solid sheet of muscle: there are holes in it through which the oesophagus and the main blood vessels from and to the heart (the aorta and inferior vena cava) must pass. The blood-vessels lie right at the back of the abdomen, just in front of the spine; but the oesophagus enters nearer the front of the diaphragm, in an opening of its own – the hiatus.

To make sure that nothing can slip upwards from the abdomen into the chest cavity alongside the hiatus – that is, between the outside wall of the oesophagus and the surrounding circular rim of the hiatus – there are powerful muscles in the hiatus's rim that hold it close to the oesophagus. These are the diaphragmatic crura (plural crurae) – a word which comes from the Latin for cross – so-called because they criss-cross around the oesophagus, keeping it tightly and effectively in place. Under normal circumstances, nothing can pass between the crural edges and the outer oesophageal surface.

This is very useful, not only for preventing a hernia, but also for ensuring that the external pressure around the last few centimetres of the oesophagus (the part that lies inside the abdomen) is high. So even if the cardia is slightly inefficient, and could possibly let stomach contents pass back into the oesophagus, this is prevented purely by the high external pressure, which effectively keeps the oesophagus collapsed until the pressure of food and peristalsis from above opens it up. In fact, this positive pressure exerted on the lower end of the oesophagus is probably the most important mechanism for preventing the back-flow of stomach contents into it. When the cardia is pushed up into the chest cavity – as happens with a hernia – and the surrounding pressure is much lower, then back-flow from stomach to oesophagus is the rule, rather than the exception.

If you have read this far without having to re-read some sections, congratulations! For by now you will have realized that what goes on in the act of swallowing, and where the oesophagus meets the stomach, is complex. And, as any biological mechanism can go wrong, it is probably best to summarize all that has been described in this chapter, to explain all the different problems which can lead to the symptoms put down to 'hiatus hernia'.

In brief: the oesophagus, in a series of muscular movements, pushes the food down through the diaphragm, where the crurae make sure that there is no unwanted return. Just below the diaphragm, the pressure on the last portion of oesophagus reinforces that function, so that the food passes into the stomach through the cardia. There, the angle between the lower end of the oesophagus and the stomach, along with the sphincter and the oblique muscles around the opening to the stomach, all combine to ensure that the food enters the stomach and cannot return. It is a perfect system – if it works! If it doesn't, there is trouble. This is explained in Chapter 3.

3

Hiatus hernia and related problems

Although this book is mainly about hiatus hernias, it has, of necessity, to cover conditions that are not strictly a form of hiatus hernia, but which for convenience are labelled as such. Many people, for example, have a hernia in another part of the diaphragm, usually next to the hiatus: strictly speaking, this is para-oesophageal or rolling hernia, but is usually called hiatus hernia for simplicity. There are subtle differences in the symptoms of hiatus and para-oesophageal hernia which were described in Chapter 1, and which will be explained later in this chapter.

However, there are also conditions, involving the oesophagus, which mimic hiatus hernia: the symptoms are very similar, but no hernia is actually present. For example, acid reflux can spread up from the stomach without there being an actual hernia; or 'pouches' in the wall of the oesophagus can fill with food or gas, and mimic a rolling hernia. These, too, will be described in this chapter, as many people with 'hiatus hernia' may well be suffering from one of them. To understand the differences between these conditions fully, you need to know a little about how the oesophagus develops in the embryo, and where the process can go wrong.

The beginnings – how trouble can develop

The oesophagus is first recognizable in the 35-day-old embryo as a millimetre-long vertical, solid cylinder with a groove along each side. As it grows the groove splits the cylinder into two tubes, the front half becoming the breathing tubes – the trachea and main bronchus – and the back half the swallowing apparatus – the oesophagus. By the time the baby is born, these two tubes are hollow and completely separate from one another, so that we can breathe and swallow without the one system interfering with the other.

Occasionally that separation is incomplete. This can lead to several conditions:

- to open tubes which join the oesophagus to the breathing system – these are called tracheo-oesophageal fistulae;
- to a blind end to the oesophagus so that it does not meet up with the stomach at all (called tracheo-oesophageal atresia);
- to a congenital oesophageal hernia, in which the cardia (explained in Chapter 2 as the junction between the oesophagus and the stomach) lies above the diaphragm, along with a portion of stomach. This is in fact an unusual form of hiatus hernia.

Surgery for new-born babies

These conditions are usually very obvious in the first few days of life, as the baby has difficulty in feeding. The main problem is vomiting or regurgitation of food. Children with tracheo-oesophageal fistulae go blue and choke at their first feed, as food spills over into their lungs – so diagnosis is usually made very quickly. Surgery must be performed, to close off the connection between the two tubes, before they have another feed.

Surgery soon after birth may also be necessary if a baby has a large hiatus hernia. This condition can sometimes mean that a large portion of the organs which should be in their abdominal cavity are inside their chest instead. This can make them very breathless and distressed, especially when lying down. Sitting them up, so that gravity causes these organs to return to the abdomen, can cause an instant improvement. However, emergency surgery is needed to return the abdominal organs to their proper positions, and to close off the hole in the diaphragm.

During the operation, whether it is for a fistula or a hiatus hernia, the surgeon ensures that the oesophagus is now long enough to reach the stomach below the diaphragm, that the diaphragm is intact, and that the cardia, below the diaphragm, is working correctly. This is essential even in the case of a tracheo-oesophageal fistula, because many such children have future trouble with a hiatus hernia. It is best if that can be prevented by the correct surgery at the time.

The early start – and the later problems

Being born with a tracheo-oesophageal fistula is much less common than being born with a hiatus hernia. Dr B. T. Johnston and his colleagues reported in 1995 on the follow-up of 192 children brought to the Royal Belfast Hospital for Sick Children between 1945 and 1972 for treatment of hiatus hernia. All the children had been admitted because of vomiting and regurgitation of food. Of those who were treated medically, two-thirds had started medical treatment (the postural chair system mentioned in Chapter 1) before the age of 6 months; the rest were treated when they were between 6 and 18 months old.

Of the 118 cases who could be traced, 94 had not had surgery, and 24 were operated upon. The interest for us now is how they managed as adults. Of those who had not had surgery, more than half of those who agreed to have barium X-rays (76 adults) still had a hiatus hernia; 43 of the 94 still had heartburn at least once a month. However, their symptoms depended to some extent on how they had responded to their medical treatment as children. Only 20 per cent of those who had responded well to postural treatment as babies still needed regular antacid treatment as adults – in contrast to 46 per cent of those who had not fared so well as children. However, even this latter group were managing fairly well: only three of them found that their heartburn was interfering with their daily activities.

Of the 24 adults in the follow-up who had needed surgery in childhood for their hiatus hernias, 14 had been over four years old when they were first seen by the hospital: by this time they already had scarring of their lower oesophagus. This suggests a strong need to give children proper treatment as early in life as possible. Eighteen of the 24 were still experiencing, as adults, heartburn at least once a month, and 13 at least once a week. Of the 20 who agreed to have a barium X-ray, 17 still had a hiatus hernia.

A crucial point made by the authors of this study was that early recognition and treatment of hiatus hernia is very important for long-term success. Of the children treated before they were six months old, 72 per cent had what was assessed as a very good outcome – as compared to 29 per cent of those whose treatment started after that time.

What about the figures for heartburn in these adults who'd had hiatus hernias as children? Superficially they look bad, with around half of them having regular heartburn. In fact, they are no worse than the figures for the general population. In five large European and North American population surveys, reported from 1976 to 1991, the proportion of 'normal' people who had heartburn (not necessarily treated by antacids) at least once a month ranged from a minimum of 20 per cent to a maximum of 44 per cent. In the Belfast group, 33 per cent were still taking antacids for heartburn at least once a month. The corresponding figures for the rest of the community, according to the surveys, ranged from 27 per cent to 32 per cent.

What did the authors conclude from their study? The main conclusion was that children with hiatus hernias should be treated as early as possible, using the postural method to begin with. If that is not successful, surgery is a second resort – but the decision to operate should be taken early, rather than later, when the oesophagus might already be scarred by constant exposure to acid.

They also concluded that children who respond to treatment do very well as adults, in that their quality of life is no different from that of the rest of the population, even if they still have their hiatus hernia. That, of course, begs the question: how many of the general population actually have a hiatus hernia without knowing it? How many of the 40 per cent or so of us who have heartburn regularly actually have a hiatus hernia?

The answer is probably academic. After all, it is the symptoms which the hiatus hernia causes, and not the hernia itself, that matter to people. If we can get rid of the symptoms, then even if a small hernia continues to exist, it does not matter. The medical argument about the proportion of the population with a hiatus hernia has been going on since 1925, when Dr L. B. Morrison, an American radiologist, found that 1 per cent of all adults surveyed had a hiatus hernia, according to his X-ray findings. This falls far short of the number who have heartburn – the major symptom of a hiatus hernia – but there must be many instances of small hernias that would not have shown up on Dr Morrison's system of tests.

The same must go for childhood. It is beginning to look as if many people have had hiatus hernias from a very early age, and that most hernias do not cause symptoms until adult life. Most respond well to the proper medical treatment, without the need for surgery. What these symptoms are, and when the decision is made to undertake surgery, rather than to offer medical treatment, will be discussed later.

Barrett's oesophagus

One condition must be mentioned here before we progress to a wider discussion of what goes wrong in hiatus hernia. This is Barrett's oesophagus.

In 1950, British surgeon N. R. Barrett wrote a paper entitled 'Chronic peptic ulcer of the oesophagus and oesophagitis'. It was published in the *British Journal of Surgery* – and since then the name Barrett's oesophagus has always been given to such cases.

People with Barrett's oesophagus have two main symptoms: they have heartburn (usually severe), and their food tends to 'come back' into the throat (regurgitation). Even when they have not been eating, they find bitter gastric secretions welling up into their mouth. If the condition continues without treatment, they develop difficulties in swallowing (dysphagia), and they also start to have a severe boring pain in the centre of the chest, which can travel through to the back. The first is a sign that scarring in the oesophagus is causing an area of narrowing (a stricture), beyond which food cannot pass easily. The second is a sign of a peptic ulcer in the oesophagus. Both are very serious signs. People in this state *must* be treated, as the next stage can be bleeding (haemorrhage) from the ulcer, or even perforation of the ulcer into the chest cavity, with all the damage that can be wrought if the lungs are exposed to the stomach's digestive juices.

In Barrett's oesophagus, the flaw is in the lining of the lower end of the oesophagus. Instead of it having the usual tough, skin-like cells which line the normal oesophagus, its lining is much more like the lining of the stomach-wall, with glands and other cells which are much more susceptible to acid attack but which do not produce adequate amounts of protective mucus. As the Barrett's oesophagus is often also associated with a hiatus hernia, it is repeatedly exposed to stomach acid and pepsin. The ensuing irritation and inflammation lead to the strictures and ulcers. There are even acid-producing cells in the Barrett's tissue itself – so it contains the mechanism of its own destruction.

Obviously, people with Barrett's oesophagus are at more danger than others with an uncomplicated hiatus hernia – and without tests it is difficult to tell, just from the symptoms, one from the other – particularly in the early stages. This is one reason why most people with relatively severe hiatus hernia symptoms are asked to undergo a series of quite unpleasant tests, to make sure of the diagnosis. These are described in Chapter 6.

Why people have a Barrett's oesophagus in the first place is still a matter of argument between experts. It was initially thought to be a congenital defect – people were born with the wrong type of lining in the lower oesophagus; but opinion has swung to the feeling that it may be an acquired condition after birth – although what causes it to be acquired is unknown.

Twenty-two years studying patients with symptoms of hiatus hernia led American surgeons J. Borrie and L. Goldwater to report that 4.5 per cent of them have a Barrett's oesophagus. Oddly, they fall into two main age-groups: children from 0 to 15 years old, and adults from 48 to 80 years old. Three times as many men as women have a Barrett's oesophagus, and there are several reports of families in which more than one member has it.

Barrett's oesophagus has been linked with cancer, but this too is a source of argument between the experts. There have been repeated, but isolated, reports of people who have both Barrett's oesophagus and oesophageal cancer. The biggest series is from the Mayo Clinic in the United States, where Dr A. J. Cameron and colleagues found, among 122 patients with Barrett's oesophagus, that 18 of them (15 per cent) also had oesophageal cancer.

This sounds very conclusive, but in more than eight years of follow-up of the remaining 104 patients, only two further cancers were found. In another series, reported by S. J. Spechler and colleagues, just two patients, out of a total of 105 with Barrett's oesophagus, developed oesophageal cancer in a follow-up of over three years. Both were heavy smokers and alcoholics who either refused to, or were unable to, stop their habits. Taking the two series together, the oesophageal cancer rate was still more than 40 times that expected of people without any known oesophageal disease – but it remains a small risk in absolute terms.

The risk is even lower if it is considered that, of the patients with Barrett's oesophagus in these studies, 85 per cent were cigarette smokers and 76 per cent were, in the words of the authors, 'addicted to alcohol'. As these two social habits are both known to raise the risks of oesophageal cancer, and may even be partly instrumental in causing Barrett's oesophagus in the first place, it is difficult to calculate the risk, if any, of cancer in the patient with Barrett's oesophagus who is a non-smoker and drinks only a little.

What these figures do mean is that if you are a smoker and heavy drinker, the first thing you must do is stop. How to do this is described in Chapter 7, which is devoted to the medical treatment of hiatus hernia.

Types of hiatus hernia

In medicine, as in many sciences, the pendulum of expert opinion swings to and fro as facts become clear and cherished theories are disproved. Fifty years ago, most experts held that most people with heartburn had a hiatus hernia: if the usual methods of identifying one did not show it, then they were probably too crude to do so – but it was accepted that one was probably present, nevertheless.

As X-ray techniques and endoscopic examination (passing a flexible fibre-optic tube into the stomach, explained in Chapter 6) became more sophisticated, and things could be seen in more detail, that opinion was gradually replaced by a view that acid could flow back (reflux) into the oesophagus without there being a hernia. The theory was that there were times when the oesophageal sphincter relaxed, and that this could allow reflux. There was also evidence, from a series of cases reported in 1968, that there were many people with hiatus hernias who had never had symptoms.

However, new evidence suggests that the relaxation of the

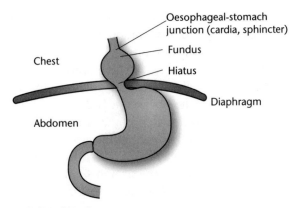

Oesophageal-stomach
junction (cardia, sphincter)

Fundus

Chest

Hiatus

Diaphragm

Abdomen

Figure 2 A sliding hernia

sphincter is not as important as was previously believed, and that most heartburn is indeed caused by a hernia. The problem lies in identifying a small hernia – it is certainly not true that the bigger the hernia the worse it is. In fact, in many cases the reverse is the case. In a 1981 study, researchers showed by using special X-ray techniques that 90 per cent of people with oesophagitis (inflammation of the oesophagus) did indeed have a hiatus hernia, but that in many cases it was small.

The sliding hernia

Figure 2 shows what happens with a sliding hernia (see Chapter 2 for an explanation of the technical terms, and of a properly working system). The basic fault is that the junction between the oesophagus and the stomach (the cardia) is not below the diaphragm, in the abdominal cavity, but in the chest. This means that all the mechanisms preventing the reflux of stomach contents into the oesophagus are lost. The oesophagus now enters the stomach at its uppermost point – at 12 o'clock instead of ll o'clock – so that there is no fundal compartment in the stomach to collect gas and to keep the pressures in the stomach low. Instead, the oesophagus enters straight into the top of the stomach with a round opening, instead of the normal angled oval, so that there is no 'flap' valve to prevent reflux. There is no diaphragmatic crura to close off the lower end of the oesophagus, and no sling mechanism to support the junction between the oesophagus and stomach. Some of the stomach is in the chest, so there are cells directly producing digestive juices in the chest, with free access to the oesophageal cells above.

It took a study using both X-rays and pressure measurements inside the oesophagus to clarify what happens during swallowing in people with a sliding hiatus hernia. F. H. Longi and P. H. Jordan showed that if people with a sliding hiatus hernia were asked to swallow some barium, and then to swallow a second time, barium that had collected in the hernia flowed back into the oesophagus as the sphincter opened to receive the second swallow.

Longi and Jordan proposed that this meant that a small amount of acid is trapped in a hernia at one swallow, and then is ejected up into the oesophagus with the next. This type of reverse movement is not present in people who have no hiatus hernia, or in people with a very large hernia.

This study (and others since which have confirmed its findings) helps to rectify what appears at first illogical – that small hiatus hernias are more likely to cause symptoms than large ones. One reason is that, according to a law of physics (Laplace's law), the pressure inside a sphere is inversely proportional to its radius: in other words, the larger the hernia, the lower is the pressure inside it. And the lower the pressure, the less is the force pushing its contents upwards. If the diameter of the hernia is much greater than that of the oesophagus (it can 'balloon' in size), no reflux can occur from hernia to oesophagus.

Also, small hernias are more likely to have a smaller opening, and retain the pressure inside them for longer, so they retain their contents for longer, and the potential for irritation is much greater. The pressure inside them is likely to be higher, so that if the sphincter is not working, or is relaxed, then back-flow is more likely to occur up into the oesophagus. Such small hernias may well have been missed by past types of investigation. They are less likely to be missed today.

How they are investigated is explained in Chapter 6, although it has to be said here that only a minority of people with hiatus hernia symptoms need such extra tests. When approaching your doctor for the first time with symptoms, you must expect them to make a diagnosis and to start you on a regimen of medical treatment and lifestyle changes before considering embarking upon intrusive investigations. You will only need these if you do not respond well to the initial therapy, and nowadays that is, thankfully, fairly rare.

The rolling hernia

About 5 per cent of all hiatus hernias are 'rollers' (or para-oesophageal hernias) rather than 'sliders'. In these cases, the fundus of the stomach 'rolls' up into the chest to lie alongside the lower end of the oesophagus (see Figure 3). The cardia remains below the diaphragm, and still works well. The angle between lower oesophagus and stomach remains in place, as do all the other mechanisms such as the sphincter and the diaphragmatic crura, so that reflux of stomach contents into the oesophagus does not take place.

This description makes it sound as if a rolling hernia is not as bad as a sliding hernia, as it does not cause heartburn or regurgitation. That is not necessarily the case, because other symptoms can be worse. For example, with a rolling hernia, quite a large portion of the stomach can be displaced into the chest: there may even be loops of intestine in the sac, and they can fill with gas.

In this case (in contrast to a sliding hernia), the larger the hernia, the worse the symptoms most definitely become. The distension of the part of the stomach which is within the chest can cause considerable pain, and a very uncomfortable bloated feeling – and the more distended it is, the more likely it is to become obstructed at

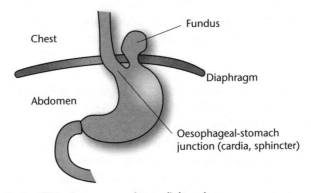

Figure 3 A rolling (para-oesophageal) hernia

the site of the opening in the diaphragm. The only way to relieve the pain and distension is by belching and vomiting: this is what wakes people in the night, to roam around the house until the symptoms can be relieved.

A para-oesophageal hernia can pose even worse problems than this: it can be so large that it takes up space normally used by the heart and lungs, so that you become extremely breathless (you feel that you cannot get a deep enough breath) and your heart begins to beat erratically. Only surgery can help at this stage.

In fact, the main treatment for all rolling hernias is surgical repair of the hole in the diaphragm through which the hernia has occurred. Even if the hole is relatively small, an early operation is now advised to prevent it from becoming suddenly bigger. It is far better to operate on a hernia under control, than to have to operate in an emergency on a person with a blocked gut inside a chest in which both the lungs and heart are in distress!

The types of operation performed for both sliding and rolling hernias are described in Chapter 9.

Oesophageal spasm – achalasia and other disorders

A description of the conditions which cause the symptoms of hiatus hernia would not be complete if it lacked what doctors know as 'functional disorders of the oesophagus'. These are not hiatus hernias but are problems with the muscles of the oesophagus, so that the normal process of peristalsis, which pushes the food into the stomach, is disturbed. There is no obvious anatomical defect in the oesophagus, diaphragm, cardia or stomach – but the lack of muscle co-ordination can create havoc with the swallowing process.

Achalasia

The most common condition is achalasia. Achalasia can start at any age, from childhood onwards. The main symptom is difficulty in swallowing (dysphagia). At first, the sufferer finds it easier to swallow liquids than solids, but after a while most food and drink seems to stick in the chest. If this state is allowed to continue, the oesophagus distends and fills with food, which can suddenly re-appear in the mouth. That is bad enough – but if it occurs during sleep, you can breathe the food in, and, if this does not choke you, it will at least cause severe irritation in the lungs. One group of achalasia sufferers find that their main symptom is repeated chest infections from minor bouts of such inhalation. In the early stages of achalasia, barium X-rays show just a bulging lower oesophagus above a short, narrowed segment which will not open. Later, the bulge becomes much bigger, and the oesophagus can eventually become like a large, soft, twisted bag full of undigested food.

Achalasia is thought to be due to the failure of the peristaltic wave to pass through the lowest segment of the oesophagus, which remains narrow and underdeveloped. There seems to be a fault in the muscles in the oesophageal wall, or in the nerves that control their contraction and relaxation, at this point. In the early stages of achalasia, the narrowed region can be stretched successfully by an instrument called a bougie or a water-filled dilator, but most cases need surgery to re-fashion the cardia so that its muscles allow the passage of food from oesophagus to stomach. This is called anterior myotomy or the modified Heller operation. This technique will be referred to again in Chapter 9.

Sadly, one occasional after-effect of the Heller operation is the start of reflux from stomach to oesophagus, so that one set of symptoms is replaced by another. However, the relief from the first is so good that the vast majority find the second trivial in comparison.

Three other oesophageal problems related to achalasia are diffuse spasm, nutcracker oesophagus and tertiary contractions.

Diffuse spasm

With diffuse spasm, the peristaltic wave is normal, but from time to time there is an extra contraction, in which the whole oesophagus goes, in effect, into cramp. The muscles along the length of the oesophagus contract, and stay contracted for minutes at a time. This causes a deep-seated central chest-pain which is often mistaken for angina or even a heart attack. (Treatment is described under nutcracker oesophagus below.)

Nutcracker oesophagus

With nutcracker oesophagus, the peristaltic wave – which is not normally an activity of which anyone is conscious – is intensified to a much higher strength and a much longer duration. It is so intense that it is felt as a very severe pain, so much so that it feels as if the cramping muscles could crack a nut inside them. X-rays taken at the time of the pain show very intense waves of contractions of the muscles in the oesophageal wall.

Both diffuse spasm and nutcracker oesophagus can be very difficult to treat. Antispasmodic drugs may help, but some people need to have regular insertion of a bougie into the oesophagus, or even an operation to cut the oesophageal muscles, before their symptoms are relieved (see Chapter 9 for a description of such surgery).

It is thought that some of these spasms (in diffuse spasm or nutcracker oesophagus) are initiated when small amounts of acid pass, by reflux, up from the stomach into the lower oesophagus. In such patients the oesophageal lining appears to be extremely sensitive to such acid, and the muscles around it respond accordingly, either with cramp or with exaggerated peristalsis that spreads through the whole length of the oesophagus.

Tertiary contractions

Tertiary contractions are a series of uncoordinated contractions of segments of oesophagus which do not aid the propulsion of food towards the stomach. They are linked in some patients with reflux, but they are also seen in older patients with no obvious symptoms. An extreme degree of tertiary spasms is called corkscrew oesophagus, in which the whole oesophagus twists on itself. Although that sounds horrendous, it hardly ever causes severe symptoms, and can be just an X-ray diagnosis seen by chance in patients being investigated for other reasons than oesophageal symptoms. Tertiary contractions rarely need any form of treatment.

4

The doctor's diagnosis

Having read the first three chapters, you will by now understand that hiatus hernia is not a single diagnosis, but a group of complex conditions with different symptoms and different underlying processes, which require different treatments. The case histories of Chapter 1, and the faults in the oesophagus, diaphragm, cardia and stomach described in Chapter 3, should have convinced you of the importance of being able to describe your symptoms to your doctor with some degree of accuracy. If you can't do that, it will take longer for your doctor to unravel the facts and match them to a diagnosis. If you wish, re-read the case histories to see how different they are – yet they all come under the diagnosis of hiatus hernia.

Keep in mind that most general practitioners will make an initial, probable diagnosis from what their patients tell them, and from a modest examination of the chest and abdomen. For most patients that is enough, and no further tests are necessary before treatment can be started. For a few, there are warning symptoms and signs which mean that the doctor must take things further, probably by referring the patient to a specialist gastroenterologist. There are times, however, when the symptoms turn out not to be due to a hiatus hernia or to oesophageal disease at all (this will be covered in Chapter 5).

Your doctor's questions

Most people, when they have plucked up the courage to face their doctor with a problem, do so because of one main symptom they have found to be intolerable or excessively worrying. Once you admit to this symptom, your doctor will be trying to link it with others, so you will be asked a series of questions designed to produce a response that will fit a particular diagnosis.

For the person with a probable hiatus hernia, the main symptom is likely to be heartburn – but as our case histories illustrate, symptoms can also range from an odd sensation of discomfort, to regurgitation of food or fluid, difficulty in swallowing, or even to bleeding. The questions you will be asked will therefore take the following pattern.

On heartburn

So you have heartburn? Can you describe it in more detail? For example, is it truly a searing or burning pain, or is it more a dull ache? Exactly where is it? Does it stay behind the breastbone, or does it move up into the jaw or into the arm (particularly the left arm)? Does it appear in the pit of the stomach, or travel into the back? Does it come on with eating? If so, does the amount of food make a difference? Or the type of food?

Your answers to these questions will already have narrowed down the options. The quality of the pain matters a lot: a burning pain points to acid in the oesophagus; a dull ache may mean the development of an oesophageal ulcer, or even pain from the heart. The distribution of the pain matters: the more widespread it is, the more extensive the oesophageal irritation, and the more likely it is that you will need more intensive treatment. Burning oesophageal pain, like angina, can spread into the jaw, arm and stomach – but if your pain is more dull and aching than burning, and extends into these areas, then your doctor will be considering angina as another diagnosis.

Heartburn-like pain with eating (particularly if it is almost imme-diate) is usually oesophageal, and the larger the meal the more likely it is to cause symptoms. But that is so for some types of angina too, so the fact that your dull ache is brought on by food does not rule angina out. The interval between starting to eat and the onset of pain, however, is usually longer for angina and for stomach ulcer – another diagnosis likely to be in the doctor's mind. Paradoxically, hunger may also bring on heartburn: that does tend to differentiate it from angina (but not from a stomach ulcer). As for the types of food most likely to bring on heartburn, alcohol, spices, raw fruit, carbonated drinks and hot drinks (especially milk-less tea) top my patients' list.

On posture

Do your symptoms get worse when you adopt any particular posture? For example, when you're stooping, bending, lying down? Do they come on when you're lifting heavy weights? How comfortable are you in bed? Do you have to sleep propped-up? Are you wakened at night with heartburn?

If you have a sliding hernia, your symptoms are likely to be greatly influenced by the position you adopt. If the pain starts when you stoop, bend over or lie down, this does strongly suggest hiatus hernia with reflux. The symptoms are often worst in bed, and many people have already found, long before they seek their doctor's help, that sleeping in a propped-up position eases the symptoms.

Most people tend to prop up the head of the bed with blocks, but that can lead to them sliding down the bed while asleep, and waking up in the small hours with heartburn because they are by this time lying flat! If you do that it is best to put a blocking board in the foot of the bed, so that your feet come up against it, to prevent you from sliding down any further. Instead, it is probably better to put blocks under the foot of the bed, and an angled support under your pillows, so that you are propped-up with your torso at an angle of around 60 degrees, and your legs at around 10 degrees, from the horizontal. Then any tendency to slide while you are asleep will be towards the head of the bed, thereby reinforcing the angle, and keeping you relatively upright while sleeping.

On 'discomfort' or other pain

Do you have pain or discomfort other than, or in addition to, the heartburn? If so, how can you best describe it? Exactly where is it? What brings it on?

The commonest pain apart from heartburn is a discomfort often described as a raw feeling or aching pain, or simply as a discomfort for which there are no more accurate words, felt mainly in the back of the throat or in the upper, central part of the chest just behind the breastbone. Although it is not usually as severe as heartburn, it is made worse by swallowing food, or hot or cold liquids. This painful swallowing can be a sign of acute oesophagitis, which may have been caused by a recent drinking bout, or over-indulgence in a curry! It does not usually last long, as acute oesophagitis settles quickly – but it is a warning against future dietary indiscretions!

A constant ache in the centre of the chest, which is not particularly made worse by food but may be worsened by hunger, may be a sign of an ulcer in an irritated oesophagus, and must be taken seriously.

On regurgitation

Do you find food or drink that you have just swallowed coming back into your mouth? This is quite different from vomiting, in which you first feel sick, and then the stomach muscles contract to heave the food up from the mouth forcefully outwards. The regurgitation of a hiatus hernia wells up without a feeling of nausea. If you do regurgitate, how soon after swallowing does it happen? Does it have the same taste as when it went down, or is there an added sour or bitter taste? Does it come with belching and gas? Are you bothered by regurgitation at night, when lying flat? Do you get breathless, and are you prone to chest infections?

The answers to these questions are important, because they can indicate how serious your problem is, and whether there is a need to operate, rather than use just medical treatment. For example, regurgitation immediately after swallowing, combined with the lack of sour or bitter taste, suggests that there is a blockage in the oesophagus – possibly a stricture from old scarring, or achalasia. A bitter or sour taste confirms that stomach contents are entering the oesophagus – so there is reflux. Belching is also an indication that stomach contents are involved. Bile – an excessively bitter-tasting green liquid in the regurgitated material – means that even the outlet of the stomach into the duodenum is not functioning properly. That means that further tests are mandatory, as there may be obstruction lower down in the gut.

Regurgitation at night is also a very important indication for further tests. If you regurgitate when you are sleeping, you can breathe some of the contents into your lungs. Two American surveys reported respectively that 60 per cent and 40 per cent of their patients with hiatus hernias had serious, chronic lung disorders such as bronchitis, asthma, bronchiectasis (in which there are multiple pockets of infection deep within the lung) and pneumonia. By 1979 the connection between night regurgitations and lung disease was being questioned. In that year, C. A. Pellegrini and colleagues studied 48 hiatus hernia patients whom they suspected were breathing regurgitated food into their lungs: only eight of them were actually doing so, five of whom had a primary lung disorder quite separate from their hernia.

The experts continue to argue about the importance of regurgitation at night. My own feeling is that if it happens to you, surgery should be strongly considered – particularly if you have any 'chesty' symptoms. I base this on the evidence of T. L. Lomasney, who found, in 1977, that surgical correction of reflux (this is explained in Chapter 9) cured or greatly improved not only the regurgitation, but also the chest problems, in the vast majority of patients.

On swallowing

Do you have difficulty with swallowing? Does it feel as if food is stuck inside your chest? How often does this happen? Is it getting worse?

The feeling that food isn't slipping down as easily as it should is very common with hiatus hernia. It can mean one of two problems. When it 'comes and goes', this is usually a sign of oesophagitis irritation of the oesophagus due to acid regurgitation. When the acid is removed with medication, the condition rapidly improves. However, if it is gradually getting worse, more frequent, and especially if it happens with every meal, a stricture must be suspected and investigated. Strictures are fixed, permanent narrowings of the oesophagus, which are usually the end-result of many episodes of oesophagitis. The repeated inflammation and healing eventually produces scars which contract and constrict the diameter of the oesophagus, and which do not open up, even under pressure. Such strictures may be at any level in the oesophagus.

Some swallowing difficulties are due to spasm of segments of oesophageal muscles. That happens in achalasia and the other muscle disorders described in the last section of Chapter 3. This also gives the feeling that food is held up deep inside the chest, but is also painful – and the feeling suddenly disappears, along with the pain, as the spasm eases off. However, in more severe forms of achalasia, the symptoms are so similar to those of an organic stricture that X-rays and endoscopy are needed to differentiate between them.

On bleeding

Have you noticed any bleeding? Is there blood in the material you bring up? What colour are your stools? Have they ever been black?

By inducing intense inflammation, oesophagitis due to acid reflux may erode into small blood-vessels just under the oesophageal lining. This can cause bleeding, which you will know about if you tend to regurgitate. The blood can appear as flecks of red or rusty brown in the liquid that appears in your mouth.

However, if you don't have this symptom, the only way you can detect regular bleeding from an irritated oesophagus is by looking at your stools. By the time blood has travelled from the oesophagus through the gut to the rectum and anus, it is changed chemically, so that it is black, rather than red. A stool containing a lot of blood is also changed in consistency, so that it is like soft tar, rather than normally formed. If you have noticed these changes, then you must tell your doctor. Black tarry stools (called melaena) are a reason for emergency admission to hospital, so that the bleeding can be stopped. You ignore them at your peril: such haemorrhages can be fatal if allowed to continue.

Not all bleeding is so obvious. The blood-loss from a chronically irritated oesophagus can be only a few millilitres a day. This will not show obviously in the stools: they may be a little darker brown than normal, but not enough to cause concern. And their consistency will not change. However, even two millilitres a day, over many months, can be enough to cause anaemia, as the body struggles to replace the loss.

Although you will not notice the loss in the stool, the modern tests for blood in the stool will pick up such small amounts. Do not be surprised, therefore, if your doctor asks for a sample of stool to test. (It is common to ask for three specimens given on three separate days, just to make sure.) You will also be asked to give blood so that your haemoglobin level and perhaps your reticulocyte count can be checked. The first is a measure of how much oxygen-carrying power your red cells have – and whether you are anaemic or not. The second is as a measure of how many young red cells you have – and therefore how hard your bone marrow is working to replace any loss. The higher the reticulocyte count, the harder the marrow is working to replace lost red blood-cells.

Very occasionally, hiatus hernia and oesophagitis can cause no symptoms – they are 'silent' – so that the first sign of trouble is a haemorrhage, which appears in the mouth or as melaena. If it is severe, it is usually caused by an ulcer in a Barrett's oesophagus (see Chapter 3). It appears that the change in the lining of the lower oesophagus which makes the Barrett's oesophagus more susceptible to ulceration also makes it less sensitive, or even insensitive, to pain. Patients with this problem usually need surgery to remove the ulcerated area, and lifelong treatment to prevent any recurrence.

On belching and bloating

Do you belch a lot? Do you feel bloated? How often does it happen?

Belching and bloating are embarrassing symptoms, but they are not a sign of anything dangerous. This is a comfort to some people, whose bloating is so intense that they fear that their stomach may burst. It won't.

It may be difficult for readers who are badly afflicted by wind to accept this, but in most cases it is caused by subconscious, excessive swallowing of air. Everyone swallows a little air from time to time, but in big gas producers, swallowing is a constant habit every few seconds – and all that can be swallowed is some saliva and a lot of air. This either has to be belched up, or passed onwards into the gut, where it eventually must be passed out at the other end of the digestive system!

The answer is to try to stop air-swallowing. That is much more difficult to do than it seems, because once you know you are doing it, the habit can become even more intense. You may need training in relaxation to help yourself.

Of course, everyone has some gas in the stomach: it is a normal part of digestion, and some air-swallowing is essential to it. If you have a hiatus hernia, this air can gather in the fundus (trapped in the chest in a rolling hernia – see Chapter 3) and cause pain and discomfort deep inside the chest. The trick is to find out how best to displace the air back into the part of the stomach that remains inside the abdomen, and be able then to belch it up. People differ in the ways they find to do this: some get up and roam the house in the middle of the night, others lie on a particular side, yet others have a favourite medicine (see Chapter 7 for a list of them).

In the meantime, if this is happening to you constantly, then you *must* make it known to your doctor, for you may have a rolling hernia that needs surgical, rather than medical, treatment to put it right. Rolling hernias sometimes have a habit of getting much bigger quite quickly, and that can lead to an emergency, as described in Chapter 3. It is far better to prevent than to experience that!

Case histories revisited

Let us now return to the patients described in Chapter 1, this time looking at their histories from their doctor's viewpoint.

Mary had a sliding hiatus hernia with oesophagitis (hence the heartburn) and eventually oesophageal ulceration (hence the central persistent pain). After a few weeks of medical management, and the supervised loss of three stones in weight, she underwent surgery to repair her hernia and to make sure that it did not return. The type of operation she had is described in Chapter 9.

Eve had a large para-oesophageal hernia that from time to time filled with food or gas. Most para-oesophageal hernias are operated upon because they can become bigger and eventually become obstructed. She was not keen on surgery, and as the symptoms had settled fairly quickly, and she had only two serious bouts of the illness separated by many years, her doctor gave her the benefit of the doubt, and managed her with drugs and lifestyle advice. He did warn her, however, that if the symptoms returned, he would strongly recommend surgery.

Harry had a moderate to large sliding hernia. He has been kept almost symptom-free on medical treatment. However, his hiatus hernia is not his doctor's only worry. The fact that he has had both gall-bladder trouble and a hiatus hernia, is a bit overweight, and (it was found at the last examination) has high blood-pressure, puts him among the 20 per cent of hiatus hernia patients with a linked disease. His doctor knows he is at higher than average risk of a peptic ulcer and of coronary heart disease, and will be watching him closely for early signs of these diseases too. However, now that he plays golf regularly, no longer smokes or crawls around under floorboards, and is losing his excess weight, he is expected to do well.

James had a Barrett's oesophagus. Happily for James the bleeding was not torrential enough to end his life before he got to hospital! He needed emergency surgery to stop the bleeding, then further surgery a few weeks later (after intense medical treatment to heal the oesophagitis), to remove the ulcer-bearing area.

Jane's diagnosis (remember she was anaemic from constant small bleeds) was not absolutely clear-cut. She might have had a stomach or duodenal ulcer – remember that one in five hiatus hernia sufferers also have an ulcer – or the bleeding could have come, by coincidence, from elsewhere in the gut. So Jane had to undergo investigations to ensure that all the possibilities were ruled out. Happily, in her case, she settled satisfactorily on long-term medical treatment for her oesophagitis. There was no need for surgery, but she promised to return to her doctor for a regular check-up, every three months initially, mainly to monitor her haemoglobin. She also accepted advice on stress management!

Billy had a torn diaphragm. He needed surgery to replace the stomach into the abdomen and to suture over the hole in his diaphragm. He was also warned about future macho challenges to his mates!

Liz's pregnancy heartburn cured itself when the baby was born.

Martha is now 81: I'm writing in 2014, three years since her emergency admission with gastric volvulus. She is fit and happy. She attends a keep-fit class for the elderly in her home village, and can bend and stretch as happily as any of her colleagues with not a hint of reflux. She is regarded as a wonder woman by the seventy-somethings who exercise with her.

Peter's hernia was also managed at home without surgery. Keeping him upright allowed his oesophagus, diaphragm and stomach to develop normally.

From all of the above cases, it is clear that there are times when doctors must consider diagnoses other than hiatus hernia as a cause of the typical symptoms. This has been touched upon in Chapter 3, where oesophageal disorders other than true hiatus hernia have been discussed. Some diseases quite apart from oesophageal disorders mimic hiatus hernia symptoms, and these are discussed in the next chapter.

5

When there is something else

Some people with hiatus hernia panic when the symptoms get worse, or when a new symptom appears for the first time. This is understandable: we all tend to look upon any pain in the chest, for example, as angina – or even a heart attack – until proven otherwise. (Angina is pain that falls short of a full heart attack.) For others, the problem is the exact opposite: they assume, because they know they have a hiatus hernia, that any new symptom is probably caused by it, and that they do not need to worry. That can be as bad for you as panicking unnecessarily, because that chest-pain this time could be a heart attack – and you need to act quickly if it is.

This chapter is therefore for both these groups of people – for want of better words, the panickers and the laid back.

'Is it a heart attack?'

The pressing question for everyone with chest-pain has to be: is it a heart attack? If you already know you have a hiatus hernia, then you are probably familiar with your particular type of chest-pain. But what happens if it changes? What are the respective chances of the new pain being caused by heart trouble or by your hernia? And could the pain be due to something else, say in the lung or the stomach?

Let us look at how your doctor will approach the investigation of your chest-pain. First, because failing to spot a heart attack has much more serious consequences than a delay in diagnosing oesophagitis, all pain behind the breastbone (called retrosternal pain), whether or not it travels into the neck or arm, is presumed to come from the heart until proved otherwise.

Doctors cannot presume that, because a retrosternal pain is caused by eating a large meal, it is due to your oesophagitis. Eating is as likely to provoke angina in a susceptible person as it is to provoke oesophageal pain in a person with a hiatus hernia – and coronary disease is more frequent in people with hiatus hernias than in the general population. It is quite common to have both oesophageal and coronary disease, and no matter how detailed a history is taken by your doctor, he or she cannot make a definitive diagnosis without doing further tests to confirm or eliminate heart disease.

If you have a new chest-pain, therefore, even if you already know you have a hiatus hernia, you will be sent for cardiac investigations. These include a straight electrocardiogram (ECG), exercise ECG testing, echocardiogram and, if the evidence supports angina, coronary angiography. (All these tests are described in my book *Living with Angina*, also published by Sheldon Press.)

Some idea of how many cases of retrosternal chest-pain are actually caused by oesophageal problems, how many are due to coronary disease, and how the two could be differentiated, was given by Drs J. R. Bennett and M. Atkinson. They studied 200 consecutive patients admitted to their hospital with such pain. In just under a quarter (23 per cent) the pain was coming from the oesophagus alone. They found that the two groups of patients – those with heart disease and those with oesophageal disease – tended to describe the quality of their pain in different ways.

Those who turned out to have heart disease spoke of their pain as 'gripping', 'vice-like' or 'tight'. Those who were found to have oesophagitis complained of 'burning'. However, the differences could not be relied upon, because there was too much overlap in the descriptions between the two groups for a definitive diagnosis to be made on quality of pain alone.

The same applied to the distribution of the pain. Both patient groups admitted to feeling the pain in the neck, jaw and arms. This was a surprise at the time of the publication, as until then doctors had assumed that pain radiating to the jaw and left arm was far more likely to come from the heart than the oesophagus. Thirty years later, this Bennett/Atkinson finding is universally accepted. Pain in the back – once held to be more likely to come from the oesophagus than from the heart – was equally common in the two patient groups. Pain in the abdomen was more of a pointer to oesophageal than to heart disease, but as it was a feature of some cases of angina, this, too, was not a definitive sign of oesophagitis.

The pain occurred more often with exercise in the heart patients and with changes in posture in the hiatus hernia patients. Breathlessness was more common in the heart patients, and regurgitation in those with hiatus hernia – but even these symptoms crossed over into the other diagnostic territories. Finally, Bennett and Atkinson stressed that chest-pain may be the only symptom of oesophageal disease such as hiatus hernia, and that it may very closely mimic angina. This is particularly true of the nutcracker oesophagus described in Chapter 3.

'Could I have both angina and oesophagitis?'

Unfortunately, the older we are, the more likely we are to have both angina and oesophagitis. Dr O. Svensson and his colleagues found that half of all their Swedish patients with coronary artery disease also had oesophagitis, or disorders such as diffuse spasms or nutcracker oesophagus.

Oesophageal disorders have also been strongly linked with a particular form of angina, Prinzmetal angina, which is now thought to be due to spasms of the muscles in the coronary arteries, rather than structural disease. Prinzmetal angina, in contrast to classical angina, occurs when you are resting, rather than taking exercise. Prinzmetal attacks are caused when the muscles in the walls of the coronary arteries go into spasm – a mechanism similar to that of the diffuse spasm disorder of the oesophagus described in Chapter 3.

In two separate studies (by Drs P. H. Ducrotte and E. L. Cattan and their colleagues) of patients with Prinzmetal disease, 58 per cent and 75 per cent respectively also had disorders of oesophageal spasm. The symptoms produced by coronary spasm and by oesophageal spasms were indistinguishable, and their cause could only be identified by tests of heart and oesophageal function, which are described in the next chapter.

In 1986, Dr G. Vantrappen coined the term 'irritable oesophagus' for those people with pain exactly like angina, but which actually stems from oesophageal disease. He described 33 patients with such pain in *The Lancet* in that year. Only 12 of them had an oesophageal spasm without reflux of acid; the rest either combined spasms with reflux or had reflux alone. When he infused a small amount of acid into the oesophagus of these patients, they all developed angina-like pain in the chest – exactly the pain for which they had been consulting their doctors. When they were given anti-reflux treatment (described in Chapter 7), their pain disappeared.

In people with true angina, instilling acid into the oesophagus has no pain-inducing effect, so this has been used as a test to differentiate between the two types of disease. True angina is more usually induced by exercise, which does not normally bring on oesophageal pain. So, if you are being investigated for central chest-pain, do not be surprised if you are given both an exercise test and an acid-instillation test.

'Could my symptoms be due to gall-bladder problems?'

We have established that the symptoms of hiatus hernia include discomfort and a feeling of fullness in the upper abdomen after meals, heartburn, belching and regurgitation of bitter fluid into the mouth. However, this array of symptoms also exactly describes what happens in gall-bladder disease – in particular, chronic cholecystitis, a long-standing inflammation of the gall-bladder.

Why do the two conditions overlap so much? It appears that when the gall-bladder is inflamed, this affects normal peristalsis at the overflow from the stomach to the duodenum, allowing bile and other digestive juices to run back up into the stomach. The mixture of the bile and the stomach's digestive juices irritates the cardia, and even if there is the smallest hiatus hernia (or even just an enlarged hiatus without a hernia), the back-flow continues up into the oesophagus.

Acid alone refluxing into the oesophagus is bad enough – but with bile as well, the irritation to the lower oesophagus is worse. Research scientists have added acid and bile, both together and separately, to pieces of human oesophagus kept alive in culture. By far the most damage was done by the two together, but bile on its own, without acid, still caused considerable irritation. This may help to explain why some people do not respond completely to medicines aimed solely at reducing the impact of acid on the oesophagus (see Chapter 7).

The problem of having both gall-bladder trouble and reflux from the stomach into the oesophagus is by no means rare. At least two British studies have shown that around half of the patients with gall-bladder disease also had oesophageal reflux. In another study (by J. R. Barker and J. Alexander-Williams), 34 per cent of patients having to have surgery for gall-bladder disease also had symptoms of oesophageal reflux. Of those who were found to have an enlarged hiatus at operation, more than 80 per cent still had oesophageal symptoms afterwards.

Barker and Alexander-Williams found that, proportionately, more women than men were cured of their symptoms by gall-bladder removal, and that the men or women with the most persistent symptoms after surgery were aged between 40 and 59 years. It seems that, if you still have symptoms after your gall-bladder has been removed, you have had two diseases – gall-bladder disease and hiatus hernia. If the symptoms stop after surgery, then your main problem has been gall-bladder disease. Your symptoms of reflux were a consequence of an irritated duodenum, stomach and oesophagus. Sadly, it sometimes takes removal of your gall-bladder to find this out!

'Might I have a peptic ulcer?'

Just as the symptoms of hiatus hernia and of gall-bladder disease are difficult, if not impossible, to tell apart, so hiatus hernia can mimic duodenal and stomach ulcer symptoms, and vice versa. In some people with hiatus hernia, the pain is mainly in the upper abdomen and radiates to the back: this is identical to some peptic ulcer pain.

As with gall-bladder disease, having both a peptic ulcer and hiatus hernia is very common. British surgeons D. Flook and C. J. Stoddard showed that acid was entering the lower oesophagus in 42 per cent of their cases of duodenal ulcer, and R. Siewart found reflux in 40 per cent of his duodenal ulcer patients. American R. J. Earlam and colleagues reported even higher figures: they saw microscopic evidence of oesophagitis in 25 of their 36 patients with duodenal ulcers.

The experts are still arguing about why people with ulcers have such a lot of oesophageal trouble: some have suggested that the sphincter muscles in the cardia are faulty, and others blame minor degrees of hiatus hernia. The jury is still out. Suffice it to say that, if you have a duodenal ulcer, it is best to assume that some of your symptoms are likely to be due to oesophageal reflux of acid, and to treat yourself accordingly. How to do that is described in Chapter 7.

'I'm often chesty – is this my hernia, or something else as well?'

I wrote in Chapter 3 that many people with hiatus hernias also have lung complications. This is because when they lie down (often in their sleep), they can inhale acid and other digestive juices that have flowed up into their upper oesophagus. Breathing in the contents of the oesophagus can cause minor symptoms, such as hoarseness or a repeated cough, but it can also lead to bronchitis, pneumonia and lung abscesses – all serious, and ultimately life threatening, conditions.

It is easy to understand that lung problems can complicate severe oesophagitis, but it appears that reflux does not need to be severe to create breathing problems. One study found that 40 per cent of patients with what was classified as 'benign oesophageal disease' (meaning a small hiatus hernia without any chronic oesophagitis or strictures) had lung problems directly due to their hiatus hernias. Many had asthma, a condition closely linked with oesophagitis by other researchers.

The actual mechanism whereby so many people with hiatus hernias also have breathing problems is not, however, as clear-cut as might be thought. Two groups of researchers found that, in 4,000 scans of swallowing, only 2 per cent of people with hiatus hernias actually breathed in their refluxed stomach contents. On the other hand, another study, which scanned 19 patients overnight, found that five of them did so. It has been shown that many patients with reflux have laryngitis, due to irritation of the upper oesophagus – and if the acid regurgitation has reached the larynx, then it is very likely to have entered the lungs.

However, there is another explanation for the connection between hiatus hernias and lung disease. There is a nerve-pathway (through the vagus nerve) which directly connects the oesophagus and the main airways (the bronchi). Put a little acid into the lower end of the oesophagus in a susceptible patient, and the bronchi will immediately constrict, giving an acute attack of asthmatic wheezing. There is no need for the patient actually to inhale any acid – the presence of acid in the lower oesophagus is enough to set it off.

This is particularly true for asthmatic children. Dr N. M. Wilson and colleagues made an overnight study of 20 children with asthma. They found that an asthma attack could be much more easily provoked when the children were lying flat and asleep, and was associated with hiatus hernias and reflux of acid into the oesophagus. The link has been proved, in that when the hiatus hernia is repaired surgically in such children, and their reflux stops, not only do their symptoms of oesophagitis disappear, but so does their asthma! In these children, anti-reflux surgery was much more successful than the use of the acid-suppressant drug cimetidine (see Chapter 7), but giving both together has been found to be even better. In another study, cimetidine has been given without surgery to asthmatic children with reflux due to hiatus hernia, and their asthma symptoms improved. The same may well be true for many adults.

'Might I have cancer?'

It is natural for people who have symptoms such as difficulty with swallowing, regurgitation and central chest-pain to fear that they may have cancer. It also has to be admitted that cancers do occur in the oesophagus, and that they may or may not be linked with long standing oesophagitis due to reflux of acid. In these days of openness and frankness about medical conditions, it is essential to understand when you should be suspicious that something other than a simple hiatus hernia may be causing your symptoms. If you do not take prompt action when these suspicions arise, you may be delaying any possible cure until it is too late.

The main symptom of an oesophageal tumour is difficulty in swallowing. It does not, as a rule, cause heartburn or pain. The first symptom may arise suddenly, perhaps when trying to swallow a particularly large chunk of food, such as a fairly tough piece of meat that has not been completely chewed. Or it may come on gradually, so that swallowing becomes slower and the food seems to take longer going down than it used to. In the later stages, there is no pleasure in eating or drinking, and you lose weight because you are not taking in any food.

However, you should have gone to your doctor long before that stage. Anyone who has any difficulty in swallowing should always see his or her doctor, who will always, in the first instance, refer the case to a specialist for X-rays and endoscopy of the swallowing mechanism.

Most of the time – and particularly when there are other symptoms of hiatus hernia, such as heartburn and symptoms caused by postural changes – the trouble is found to stem from a stricture. This is a narrowing of the oesophagus due to old scar-tissue, which in turn has been caused by years of exposure to acid.

One relatively rare cause of difficulty with swallowing goes by at least three different names: it may be called sideropaenic dysphagia, or Patterson-Brown-Kelly syndrome, or Plummer-Vinson syndrome. (The name the doctor uses depends on which medical school he or she attended!) Whatever it is called, it affects women aged between 30 and 60 years old, and has three features: severe anaemia, a chronic inflammation of the tongue, and choking when trying to swallow solid food.

The swallowing difficulty in this condition starts because there is oesophageal spasm, which is limited to the upper half of the oesophagus, but which eventually becomes a stricture, when the difficulty in swallowing becomes much worse. On looking down the throat, a web can be seen stretched across it, at the level of the larynx. If this is neglected, cancer can develop in the area of this web, so it should be seen urgently. The treatment is to give iron to counter the anaemia and to remove any stricture. Follow-up includes blood tests to ensure that the anaemia is not returning, and examinations to ensure that no malignant change is occurring.

Achalasia, strictures and Patterson-Brown-Kelly syndrome apart, swallowing difficulties may be caused by tumours in the oesophagus.

Some oesophageal tumours are benign leiomyomas – over-growths of oesophageal wall-muscle that project into the passage, interfering with the food passing through its lower end. Leiomyomas are usually easily removed through an endoscope (an instrument to remove them can be passed down the flexible, hollow endoscope).

Cancers of the oesophagus are a disease of older age: 75 per cent of oesophageal cancers occur in people over 60 years old. It attacks three times as many men as women. About half of all cancers of the oesophagus arise in the middle third of its length, and about 30 per cent in its lower third, suggesting to most experts that con-stant exposure to reflux of acid from the stomach may contribute to the cause. (Although the lower third is more exposed to acid, the middle third is thought to be more sensitive to acid-provoked cancerous changes.) So repairing a hiatus hernia and stopping the oesophagus from being awash with acid may well prevent many cancers – a good reason for sticking strictly to one's doctor's advice and treatment. This is particularly true if you have a Barrett's oesophagus (see Chapter 3), which is associated with a higher than normal incidence of cancer.

Proof that looking after yourself may, by curing oesophagitis, prevent cancer is suggested by a study by R. Kuylenstierna and E. Munch-Wickland, written up in the *Journal of Cancer* in 1985. They looked back on the case histories of 163 patients with oesopha-geal cancer: 10 per cent of them had had oesophagitis. Of the 51 patients with lower oesophageal cancer, 13 (25 per cent) had had oesophagitis. There were no cases of oesophagitis among the 47 with upper oesophageal cancer (the other 65 had cancer of the middle third of the oesophagus). It seems clear from these figures that chronic oesophagitis can precede cancer of the lower oesopha-gus if it is not kept under control or even eradicated.

This whole chapter can be summarized in a few sentences. Hiatus hernia and oesophagitis are inextricably linked and give rise to many different symptoms and collections of symptoms. These can be confused with the symptoms of other conditions such as heart disease, gall-bladder disease, peptic ulcers, bronchitis and asthma, and cancer. Making a definitive diagnosis of hiatus hernia with reflux and oesophagitis is often (almost always, in fact) impossible without conducting some tests. So, if you are seeing your doctor for the first time with symptoms typical of hiatus hernia, you will almost certainly be referred to a specialist gastroenterological clinic for such tests.

These tests are described, along with the reasons for them, in the next chapter.

6

Tests for hiatus hernia and reflux

Once your doctor suspects you have a hiatus hernia he or she will take one of two decisions: either to make the diagnosis on the information you have given, plus a brief examination; or to ask a specialist gastroenterologist to do further tests to make sure.

If your diagnosis is made without such a referral, this is not neglect. The tests take up valuable consultant time and are very expensive in themselves – so, if the diagnosis can be made from the symptoms alone, this is a great saving. In these times of health costs rapidly spiralling upwards, such savings are vital. Doing without tests also allows treatment to be started earlier, and if the symptoms respond to the initial treatment, this is in effect a practical confirmation of the diagnosis. It is also much more pleasant for the patient – some of the tests can be uncomfortable, if not even distressing.

Symptom-score systems

However, any diagnosis, even one made from symptoms alone, should be based on objective judgement, and not on a vague basis. Several groups of gastroenterologists have therefore set up symptom-score systems to determine how severe the condition is, and how they might best manage the condition.

Here it must be said that the most important aim of investigating people with hiatus hernia symptoms is not to find out the size of the hernia (you can have a large hernia without symptoms, while a small hernia can cause huge problems). Instead, the priority is to determine the severity of the oesophagitis that has been caused by the hernia, and the best way to reverse its effects. It is the oesophagitis, after all, that causes the heartburn and pain, and that can lead to future oesophageal ulcers, strictures, bleeding and even perforation.

Table 1 Scoring system for symptoms of oesophagitis
(from DeMeester *et al.*)

Symptom	Grade	Description
Heartburn		
None	0	No heartburn
Mild	1	Occasional episodes
Moderate	2	Reason for visit to doctor
Severe	3	Enough to interfere with daily life
Regurgitation		
None	0	No regurgitation
Mild	1	Occasional episodes
Moderate	2	Predictable on moving position or straining
Severe	3	Associated with night-time cough or pneumonia
Swallowing difficulty (dysphagia)		
None	0	No dysphagia
Mild	1	Occasional episodes
Moderate	2	Needs a drink to clear it
Severe	3	At least one episode of obstruction needing medical treatment

The aim is to cure the oesophagitis. If that means just protecting the oesophagus from acid, then so be it. If it means surgery to repair the hernia, and therefore stop the reflux of acid into the oesophagus, then that has to be decided upon too. The symptom scores are therefore a measure of oesophagitis, rather than of the hernia itself, and they help the doctor to make the decision on how to treat a particular patient.

Two scoring systems are in general use. The first was developed by Dr T. R. DeMeester and his colleagues. It takes three separate symptoms of oesophagitis and grades each of them according to their severity on a scale of 0 to 3 points (see Table 1). The grades are very specifically described, so that people with similar scores

Table 2 Scoring system for oesophagitis (from Jamieson and Duranceau)

	One point	Two points	Three points	Four points
Frequency	Less than once a month	More often than once a month, but less often than weekly	More often than once a week, but less often than daily	Every day
Duration	Less than 6 months	More than 6 months; less than 24 months	More than 24 months; less than 60 months	More than 60 months
Severity	Nuisance value only	Spoils enjoyment of life	Interferes with living normally	Worst possible symptoms

The score for frequency is added to that for duration and the sum is multiplied by that for severity. This gives a minimum score for each symptom of 2 and a maximum of 32: the case is classified as mild if the score is in the range 1–7, moderate 8–15, marked 16–23 and severe 24–32.

have a similar severity of disease. This is important not just so that treatment can be decided on a standard assessment, but also so that clinical trials of new treatments can be fairly assessed and the results subjected to good statistical evaluation.

An alternative to this system was developed by Drs G. G. Jamieson and A. C. Duranceau. They assigned to each symptom a series of points according to the severity, frequency and duration of symptoms – the higher the score, the more severe the problem. Table 2 shows how this system works: it can be used for each symptom (heartburn, swallowing difficulties including pain, regurgitation, bleeding and chest problems); the scores for each symptom are added together to give an overall score.

Once the history has been taken, the examination completed and the provisional diagnosis made, the next step (if it is decided to investigate further, and not just to start treatment) is to plan the tests to be done.

The tests measure four areas of oesophageal function:

● its ability to swallow;

- the presence of any refluxed stomach material;
- any damage to the inner layer of oesophageal lining;
- the response of the lowest part of the oesophagus to acid.

The tests involved X-rays, endoscopies, biopsies and other tests to assess the oesophageal physiology (such as manometry to assess the pressure within the oesophagus). These will all be described in turn.

X-ray tests

X-ray examination is usually the first test. A straight X-ray of the chest can sometimes show a gas bubble within the stomach well above the diaphragm, confirming a hiatus hernia – but this can be difficult to see, and depends on there being air in the stomach at the time of the X-ray. So 'contrast' X-rays are used to make things much clearer.

The usual technique involves a barium drink, which the patient swallows while the radiologist watches the moving film. The changing shape of the lump of barium passing down the oesophagus can show up problems of mobility (such as achalasia and spasm), the presence of reflux through the cardia, and can even indicate inflammation in the lower oesophagus. Such barium-swallows have shown that many patients with reflux oesophagitis also have a much slower clearance of barium from the lower end of the oesophagus into the stomach.

However, a barium-swallow alone is not always a reliable indicator of reflux and oesophagitis. For example, one study revealed that there was a reflux on a barium-swallow in 20 per cent of patients who were later found not to have any oesophagitis, and there was no reflux in 35 per cent of people who had moderate and severe oesophagitis. To make the test more accurate, another study looked at the reflux produced when patients lay on their left side and were given the barium and some water to drink. They were then asked to turn to their right sides and given some food (bread and paté). The aim of this was to expose the maximum opening of the cardia, from stomach back to the oesophagus, to the pressures of both food and gravity: if there is reflux, it should show in this position. This study found a connection between reflux and oesophagitis in 15 out of 26 patients with symptoms. In all, 20 had food-stimulated reflux, and 23 had oesophagitis.

Do not be surprised, therefore, if when you have your barium swallow you are moved around from side to side: your radiologist is trying to see if you have any reflux. If you do, its extent will be graded by how far it travels up your oesophagus – and your treatment will be planned accordingly.

Two refinements on the usual barium-swallow have been introduced in the last few years. One is a double contrast technique, which involves the patient swallowing some barium very quickly; the oesophagus is then distended with gas from a fizzy powder (you may be asked to swallow air instead). With the other technique, you are asked first to swallow about a tablespoon of alkaline solution, then about half a cupful of barium, a tablespoon of an acid solution and three drops of a 'bubble-breaker'. This shows up the lining of the lower oesophagus in great detail, even to the extent of highlighting small ulcers in its surface. It gives the radiologist a very accurate picture of how much reflux there is, and the extent of the damage it has done to the oesophagus. Both of these techniques have shown that many people have a hiatus hernia without actually having oesophagitis, but that if you have oesophagitis, then there is almost always a hiatus hernia with acid flowing freely back through the cardia.

Endoscopy and biopsy

The flexible fibre-optic endoscope has made a huge contribution to our knowledge of medicine in recent years, and nowhere more so than in the investigation of hiatus hernias and oesophagitis. An endoscope is a fully flexible tube inside which is a bundle of glass fibres through which the operator can see very clearly what is going on inside the throat, oesophagus and stomach. It also allows instruments to be passed along its length so that biopsies (pieces of tissue) can be taken for tests, in full view of the operator.

The endoscope is passed, under local anaesthetic, into the oesophagus. It may sound horrendous to have such a procedure without a general anaesthetic, but the sedative makes you so drowsy beforehand that you hardly feel the discomfort, and will have very little memory of it afterwards.

Endoscopy gives its operator a clear, magnified view of what is happening over the whole length of the oesophagus, the cardia and the stomach. It is used for diagnosis, to assess the severity and extent of oesophagitis, and for biopsies (explained below). An endoscopy can also be used to relate the site of the cardia (the junction between oesophagus and stomach) to the level of the diaphragm: this site is clearly seen as the Z-line, a sharp difference in appearance of the surface as oesophageal tissue becomes stomach tissue.

Endoscopy is still a relatively young technique, so it is not surprising that the experts still disagree on how to assess the severity of oesophagitis. They have, however, partly agreed on a classification of oesophagitis which helps them to decide on how to proceed with treatment. Grade I oesophagitis means that the only sign of inflammation is some redness and a little friability; Grade II indicates that there are some superficial ulcers (something like mouth ulcers); Grades III and IV show many more, and deeper, ulcers, with strictures or shortening. Barrett's oesophagus is Grade IV.

As a rule of thumb, people with the lower grades of oesophagitis are usually given medical (rather than surgical) treatment; those with higher grades are at more risk of bleeding and other complications, and are likely to be treated more intensively with more powerful drugs, and to be seen more often. If they have a hiatus hernia along with their higher grade oesophagitis (which is usually the case), they will be put on the urgent waiting-list for repair.

Just looking at the oesophageal lining does not always give a definitive diagnosis: biopsies to confirm inflammation at the microscopic level may be needed. This means that the endoscope is adapted to take several tiny pieces of tissue from different, suspicious-looking areas at each endoscopy session. Taking biopsies does not cause pain. Scientists have agreed on the microscopic appearances that confirm oesophagitis in a biopsy sample, so taken together, the appearance of the oesophagus through an endoscope and the appearance of a biopsy sample through a microscope make for a very accurate diagnosis.

Manometry – measuring pressures

Not all hiatus hernia sufferers have oesophagitis. The case histories in Chapter 1 show that the problem for some is not heartburn, but pain from oesophageal spasm, or from the bulk of a rolling hernia in the chest. Through an endoscope such cases look normal. Their problem is that the pressures inside the oesophagus during spasms, or when the herniated stomach is full of food or gas, can be very abnormal, and measuring these pressure-swings can be a great help both in diagnosis and in assessing treatment.

To investigate such patients, manometry (pressure measurement) is of great value. There are two systems: both use thin catheters (one system uses a hollow tube, the other a solid one) which are passed through the nose into the oesophagus and stomach. Both systems measure the pressures above, within and below the sphincter, and the pressure-waves produced in peristalsis.

Although manometry is not useful in diagnosing oesophagitis, it can establish that a patient has one of the muscle (or motility) disorders such as achalasia, diffuse spasm or nutcracker oesophagus. However, a single patient can have both types of oesophageal disorder. In one study of 102 patients with diagnosed oesophageal acid reflux due to hiatus hernia, manometry showed that six also had achalasia, four had diffuse spasm and two had a nutcracker oesophagus. When planning their treatment, whether it is surgical or medical, it is important to take both conditions into account: surgery to repair a hernia in such patients may not cure their symptoms.

It must be said here that manometry is a very specialized investigation which will always be confined to a small proportion of patients with particular problems. The same can be said of the next investigations – provocation tests.

Provocation tests

Sometimes the description of a symptom such as heartburn is unusual. It may not be described as burning, it may appear in an unusual place, or it may not relate to food or hunger – yet the doctor may suspect that it is caused by acid reflux from stomach to oesophagus. In any of these cases, an acid provocation test may be carried out.

Its aim is simply to see whether putting a little acid into the lower oesophagus provokes the symptom of which the patient is complaining. That is not as bad as it sounds, as only a little acid is used, and many precautions are taken to ensure that no damage is done.

The Bernstein test

Three provocation tests are in current use: the Bernstein test, the acid clearance test and the standard acid reflux test. As with other aspects of hiatus hernia investigations and diagnosis, the experts do not agree on their relative usefulness.

In the Bernstein test, you sit in a chair and a thin catheter is passed through your nostril down into your lower oesophagus. As with all such catheter tests, you may choke a little as the end passes your larynx, but once the tube is in place you hardly notice it. Once you are settled, a little saline (salt solution) is passed through the catheter for about 15 minutes. At some time after this, without your being told, the saline is replaced by an acid solution for about 30 minutes. If the symptoms do not appear during this time, it can be assumed that they are not caused by acid reflux. If they do appear, the acid is immediately replaced by saline. This usually relieves the pain quite quickly, at least within 20 minutes. Only a few people report that the pain lasts longer. As soon as the test is finished you are given an antacid.

A positive Bernstein test only shows that your oesophagus is sensitive to acid: its main use is to help sort out the cause of a pain in patients whose symptoms are not the run-of-the-mill ones typical of oesophagitis or hiatus hernia.

The acid clearance test

The acid clearance test is also performed with the patient in a sitting position. Usually carried out just after manometry, it is done with the pressure-measuring catheter still in place. You will be asked to swallow another fine tube, this time with an acid-measuring electrode at the end. A little acid is passed into the lower end of the oesophagus through the manometry catheter, and you are asked to swallow every 30 seconds until the acid no longer registers with the electrode. The acid clears after three swallows in normal subjects: it can take many more in people with oesophagitis.

The acid reflux test

The standard acid reflux test measures whether you can keep acid, which has been introduced into the stomach, out of the oesophagus. This time, acid is put into the stomach via a catheter, and readings from the acid-measuring electrode are taken on either side of the cardia. In people with no reflux, the acid disappears less than one centimetre above the cardia; in people who have reflux, the acid is still registering for some distance up into the lower oesophagus. During this test you are asked to cough, to take deep breaths, and to strain as if you are lifting a heavy weight, in four positions. The test is positive if acid passes through into the oesophagus on at least two occasions in the 20 tests and positions. This test identifies people with moderate to severe reflux, but it can only be used along with the results of the other examinations as a guide to treatment: it is not accurate enough to be used alone.

Acid monitoring

Because their results are less reliable than we would wish, many gastroenterologists now use pH monitoring as their main test for reflux. The pH scale measures acidity and alkalinity: it ranges from less than 1 (extremely acid) to under 14 (extremely alkaline), with neutral being a pH of 7.

The technology of pH monitoring is changing very fast, so that in the few months between my writing this and its publication, what I write about the pH sensors may well already be out of date. However, the principles remain the same. The aim is to leave a pH monitor for 18–24 hours in the lower oesophagus, to record everything happening during that time. One system uses radio telemetry, allowing you to go home, so that the pH changes can be recorded during your normal, everyday life.

As with other aspects of hiatus hernia and its complications, the experts disagree on what constitutes abnormality and its severity. Most feel that a pH of 4 or less in the oesophagus is abnormal, but debate continues as to how long it should be at that level, and under what circumstances, before it is considered serious. However, 'normal' levels have been established: in Professor Alfred Cuschieri's unit in Dundee, 24-hour pH monitoring of 50 volunteers with no symptoms showed very few occurrences of a pH below 4, especially when they were lying down, and extremely few of these occurrences lasted for five minutes or more.

The most sensitive test for assessment of reflux is 24-hour pH monitoring. Shortened to 12 hours, the test is still reasonably accurate, and many hospital departments have shortened it further, to the three hours after a meal, with little if any further loss of accuracy. The shorter tests are cheaper and more convenient, but the 24-hour test remains, according to Professor Cuschieri, the 'gold standard' because it traces the evolution of reflux over a whole, typical day and night.

An 18–24-hour monitoring test has proved very useful in children: tiny electrodes are used, and most children tolerate it reasonably well, considering that it involves inserting tubes down the throat. American paediatric gastroenterologists have shown that it is a reliable basis for deciding upon surgery in infants.

Radio-isotope scans

The newest test involves asking you to swallow material containing a tiny amount of radiation, and following what happens with a 'gamma camera' as the food is propelled down the oesophagus into the stomach. You are asked to sit upright, and chew a dessertspoonful of poached egg-white in which there is a tiny amount of radioactive technetium (a substance that very rapidly loses its radioactivity, so it can do no harm).

You are then asked to swallow the egg-white in a single gulp, and to keep swallowing every 20 seconds thereafter. The gamma camera records what is going on for four minutes. The time it takes for all the egg to pass into the stomach is less than 15 seconds in a normal oesophagus; it can take much longer than this if you have a hiatus hernia. Professor Cuschieri's team have identified five different patterns of passage of food down the oesophagus and into the stomach from this test, and can relate them to the clinical symptoms. One of these patterns, of course, is normal. Other patients show:

- oscillation, in which the egg-white bounces down and up the oesophagus;
- non-clearance, in which the egg-white does not enter the stomach within the four minutes;
- step-delay, in which it is held up in the middle or lower third of the oesophagus;
- non-specific, in which the flow is abnormal, but does not fit into a particular pattern.

Oscillation is the typical pattern in achalasia, and Professor Cuschieri recommends this test for screening patients suspected of having this or one of the related oesophageal motility disorders.

Radio-isotope scans are often used for children, in which case the material is given in fruit-juice or milk, and the scan continues for up to an hour. As there is no tube to be swallowed or inserted, children tolerate it much better than the other tests, so it is being increasingly used as a screening test before the decision on how to treat the child is taken.

Treatment, for children and adults, has three aspects: management of one's own lifestyle, medication and surgery. They will be discussed in the next three chapters.

7

Managing your own hiatus hernia

The firm aim of all treatment for hiatus hernia is to reduce the symptoms. Whether these are caused by oesophagitis, leading to heartburn and regurgitation, or by the presence of a large mass of stomach in the chest, leading to pain, bloating and swallowing difficulties, the need is the same: to keep the stomach and cardia below the diaphragm, and to minimize the possibilities for reflux.

This needs an effort from you, as well as your doctors. You need to understand what to avoid and how to promote a healthier relationship between your oesophagus, diaphragm and stomach. It may need several changes (some drastic) in your lifestyle to make a real difference.

Posture, position and keeping fit

First and foremost, you must avoid postures and actions which cause reflux and increase the size of the hernia through the hiatus. Above all, that means any action which increases the pressure inside the abdomen, pushing the cardia up through your hiatus. Bending over is the obvious action that immediately springs to mind. When you bend, your abdominal-wall muscles contract, increasing the pressure inside the abdominal cavity. If you have a larger hiatus than normal, it is easy for that pressure to force the upper part of the stomach through into the chest, thereby flooding the lower oesophagus with acid. Heartburn is the inevitable response.

So until your hiatus hernia is mended and your oesophagitis has healed, do not bend over. This is a good excuse for all those awkward jobs you don't really like, such as weeding the garden, or clearing out bottom drawers! But it also rules out some sports, such as bowls or curling.

Postural changes are not the only means of making the abdominal muscles contract (and thus further damage the oesophagus):

lifting heavy weights (such as the weekly shopping, or a bucket of coal or logs), or pushing a loaded wheelbarrow or lawnmower, are others. Straining to pass a constipated stool is yet another, so do modify your diet (if necessary) to keep your bowel-movements regular and your stools soft. Doing weight-training can also be a problem; any explosive sport, such as weight-lifting or throwing, or even squash (we push up the pressure inside the abdomen when we hit a ball while holding our breath) can set off symptoms.

Keeping fit is highly recommended, but do so with exercises in which you keep breathing steadily, such as walking, running and dancing. Swimming is fine for people who swim semi-upright, but it can pose problems for those who swim relatively flat, and especially when the stroke demands lying on the right side. Diving is not recommended! Cycling is fine, as long as you don't have to crouch over the handlebars.

Lying down, even with your abdominal muscles relaxed, can promote a back-flow of acid into the oesophagus, or the displacement of the stomach upwards in a rolling hernia – so try to keep your chest above your abdomen at all times, even when you are sleeping. With a mild hiatus hernia and few symptoms, all you may need is an extra pillow or two. If you find this is not enough, then try the blocks under the foot of the bed and a pillow support as described in Chapter 4. If you put blocks under the bed-head, make sure you can't slip down the bed when you are sleeping.

Eating

How you eat matters more than what you eat. In the past, people with hiatus hernias were advised to eat various weird and wonderful diets, the main components of which were milk, biscuits and steamed white fish. There was absolutely no scientific basis for these diets – all they did was tend to make things worse by causing sufferers (from the diet, that is!) to gain weight. People were also advised not to eat or drink 'acid' foods, such as citrus fruits and juices. This was a complete misunderstanding of digestion: the acid in our stomachs does not relate in any way to the amount of fruit of any kind that we eat.

It is important, however, to time your meals correctly, and to eat the right quantities at each meal. If you eat a small amount every two hours, your stomach settles down to produce a small, constant amount of acid throughout the day. This acid is used up in digesting your small meals. It is far less likely to provoke oesophagitis than the usual three large meals a day, which stimulate the stomach to secrete large volumes of acid and pepsin, much of which can overflow into the oesophagus.

In addition, the larger the volume of food you pack into your stomach, the more likely it is to be displaced up into your chest, especially if you feel drowsy afterwards and are keen to put your feet up! On the other hand, don't go to bed at night on a completely empty stomach: a small glass of milk and a biscuit can help then to neutralize any acid produced during the first few hours of sleeping. Don't eat or drink more than this: a larger meal just before lying down (or for that matter just before exercise) is likely to promote symptoms by distending the stomach and increasing the pressure within it. That can lead to regurgitation of food through the cardia into the oesophagus – the last thing you need at night.

If you do feel a particular item of food causes pain, then avoid that food in the future. However, there is no reason to become faddy with your food, or to restrict what you eat generally. Keep in mind that everyone needs to eat a wide range of foods with the proper amounts of fats, carbohydrates, proteins, vitamins, minerals and water to remain healthy, and that many restricted diets are deficient in one or another of them.

Obesity

Just as important as the instructions about eating is advice about weight. Do not let yourself become overweight, and if you are overweight, do lose the extra pounds. Many hiatus hernia sufferers are several kilograms – or even stones – overweight; they often lose their symptoms completely when they return to the normal weight for their height.

This is particularly true if you have apple-shaped rather than pear-shaped obesity. The difference between the two is obvious once you recognize the terms: apple-shaped people put on their extra fat around their middle; pear-shaped people have big bottoms and hips. If you are apple-shaped, much of your fat is laid down inside the abdomen, so that it competes with the stomach for room. If the hiatus is larger than normal, the stomach is pushed up and through it. Take away the extra abdominal fat, and you leave room for the stomach to find its proper place. However, if you are pear-shaped, do not let what is written above about apple-shaped people make you complacent. People with pear-shaped obesity often find that losing weight helps their hiatus hernia symptoms enormously. Why this should be is not known: suffice it to say that the reason for the improvement does not matter so much as the result!

Losing weight is not easy for anyone – but it is more difficult for hiatus hernia sufferers than most, because they often find that dairy products and biscuits are the best way to ease their pain. These foods also happen to be full of fat-inducing calories. If you are overweight and find yourself going for the fridge each time you feel pain, make a diversion towards the medicine cabinet instead, and take a little antacid, instead of milk. Once you start losing weight you should find yourself making fewer trips to either destination.

The best way to lose weight is to eat a little less of what you normally eat, and exercise a little more, in a way that you enjoy. Don't try any crash diets: they never work permanently (no one sticks to them permanently, and most dieters have a massive rebound to an even higher weight than before), and they can be very sore on oesophagitis. Irregular meals and imbalanced eating can increase the amount of acid in the stomach – and worsen your oesophagitis. And don't go out and buy an exercise machine: very few people have the discipline to keep using one in their home, on their own. It is a good idea to join a group of like-minded people: you can gain a lot of confidence when you start to lose weight, and make friends while you do so.

Drinking and smoking

The oldest medical cliché is that we can keep healthy if we do everything in moderation. Sadly, this just isn't so for people with hiatus hernia who like a drink and a smoke!

Alcohol relaxes the cardia, so it can actually promote reflux. In the form of neat spirits, it directly irritates the lower oesophagus, especially one affected by oesophagitis. So avoid spirits completely. Remember that this advice comes from a Scot living in a whisky-distilling district, so it is given only after much deliberation and even anguish! The good news is that wines and ales are less likely to be a problem, as long as they are restricted to a glass or two in any one day. If you are drinking up to the legal limit for driving (which is in any case too high), you are probably drinking too much.

I have no such good news for cigarette smokers. If you smoke only one cigarette per day, then that is one too many. There are dozens of reasons for not smoking – among them the 100,000-plus early deaths directly due to smoking in Great Britain every year – and they are certainly applicable to hiatus hernia sufferers.

To start with, cigarette smoking lowers the pressure across the cardia, so it causes more reflux. Secondly, it directly irritates the oesophageal surface, so that it worsens oesophagitis. If that were not enough, it also delays the healing of any ulcer, so it can make bleeding and perforation more likely – especially in severe cases, such as in Barrett's oesophagus. Finally, cigarette smoking pro-motes cancer, so it is a crazy habit for people in whom the risk is already raised, however slightly, because they have oesophagitis or a Barrett's oesophagus.

Stopping smoking

If you have had difficulty in stopping smoking, or if you think that the smoking warning does not apply to you, or that you are willing to continue taking the risk, then mull over the next few paragraphs. If you heed them, they may save your life.

In the 1980s I, like many other doctors at the time, advised people that they could stop in one of two ways. They could do it gradually, over several weeks, or they could stop suddenly, all at once. Now I'm convinced that the latter is by far the better way.

It's called the General de Gaulle method, because he announced to the whole French nation, on television, that he had stopped smoking. After that, he could hardly light up in case a member of the press or a political opponent saw him and exposed him as a fraud or backslider! Most of us could do the same. We may not be as famous as the General, but we all have a circle of friends whose respect we wish to keep, and we could do something similar in front of them. Today the anti-smoking climate will ensure their sympathy and support, rather than sneers or sniggers.

I advise people to take all the cigarettes they possess, in pockets, handbags, at home or elsewhere, to scrunch them up and throw them in the bin or on the fire. They should then resolve never to buy another cigarette, and always to say 'No' immediately, without even thinking about it, to anyone who offers them one. If they do not wish to argue with smoking friends, a non-smoking sticker in the car and on the front window of their home can help.

People who contemplate stopping smoking suddenly often fear withdrawal symptoms, such as agitation, irritability, sleeplessness and nervousness. They do not need to: often there are no withdrawal symptoms. People who have to give up smoking for serious medical reasons, such as lung cancer or heart disease, hardly ever have withdrawal symptoms, probably because they realize fully why they have to stop. The same applies to anyone with hiatus hernia and oesophagitis, and particularly if they have Barrett's oesophagus. Smoking can kill, through a bleed or a perforation because an ulcer has failed to heal, or because chronic oesophagitis has turned into cancer. This is as serious as a health problem can get, and once the truth hits home, smokers then find it easy to stop.

Once you have stopped, you may still have the desire to smoke, but that will subside before long, and your new feeling of wellbeing, caused by the elimination from your body of carbon monoxide, nicotine and tars, will take over. You may well find, too, that the pain from your oesophagitis is much less, as the raw oesophageal lining begins to heal.

If you must take your mind off cigarettes, then chew low-calorie gum, or a piece of carrot or celery. Get friends to support you in your efforts.

If you can't stop the first time, try again. Many people find that they have to stop several times before they manage to do it permanently. Try acupuncture or hypnotherapy if you wish – though they do not have any magical properties: they cannot overrule weak willpower. Don't try nicotine chewing-gum or patches, because they keep up the supply of nicotine to your irritated oesophagitis – nicotine being the agent that prevents healing! It is the most powerful constrictor of arteries, and you need good blood flow to your oesophagus if it is to heal.

A good viewpoint to take, if you find stopping difficult, is to understand that over the years, you have used it as a crutch in times of stress. Obviously it is not a helpful crutch because it in no way changes the cause of your stress. So, if you must, replace it with another crutch, which could be beneficial to your health – that can be anything, even starting to enjoy fruit again. Most smokers do not enjoy fruit or vegetables because their taste-buds are so damaged by the smoke. When you stop smoking, your sense of taste comes alive again, and you can expand the variety of food you enjoy eating. This will not only benefit your general health, but help your oesophagus to heal too.

This is an ideal time to take up a new hobby, and meet new friends. If you have been a regular smoker, your regular haunts are likely to have a smoky atmosphere: so change your social life. Avoid places where most people smoke, and be on guard against the offer of that first cigarette. One quickly leads to another, and you will soon be on track to repeated oesophagitis and chest-pain. Whether the chest-pain is coming from your hiatus hernia or from your heart will again be your worry – and, to a great extent, your fault.

If you have oesophagitis and you smoke, you owe it to yourself and your family to stop. Take heart from the fact that you are not alone. Several million Britons have given up tobacco during the last 15 years. Fewer than one in three British adults now smokes. By stopping you are simply joining the sensible majority. You are also making big changes in your own physiology. Here is a list of the practical benefits of stopping smoking. It may help you in your resolve!

Within 20 minutes of stopping:
- Your blood-pressure decreases to the normal range;
- Your pulse slows down to the normal rate;
- The circulation in your fingers and toes, and in your oesophagus, begins to open up.

After eight hours:
- Carbon monoxide levels in the blood return to normal;
- Oxygen levels in the blood return to normal.

After one day:
- Your chances of a heart attack have already diminished.

After two days:
- Your senses of smell and taste are heightened;
- Your coronary arteries are much wider;
- There is much better blood-flow to your oesophagus;
- Your blood is much less likely to clot.

After three days:
- Your airways have opened up;
- You are breathing more easily;
- Your heart is more efficient and less strained.

After two weeks to three months:
- Walking is easier;
- You can exercise for much longer;
- Your circulation is much improved.

After nine months:
- Your lungs are free of tars;
- You no longer have a morning cough.

After five years:
- Your annual lung cancer death-risk has dropped from 137 to 72 per 100,000.

After ten years:
- Your annual lung cancer death-risk has dropped to 12 per 100,000;
- You are at much less risk of dying from cancer of the mouth, pharynx, oesophagus, bladder, kidney or pancreas.

Surely, if you have been a smoker until now, these facts will have persuaded you to stop. So enjoy the fact that you are now a non-smoker. You have probably prolonged your life by many years through making that decision.

However, self-management alone may not clear your symptoms. The next chapter explains how medical treatment can help you further.

8

Medical treatment of hiatus hernia

Many people who have just been told that they have a hiatus hernia are worried by the prospect that this must eventually mean an operation. This anxiety can be dispelled in the vast majority of cases. A combination of the self-management and lifestyle changes mentioned in Chapter 6 with a simple drug regimen is usually all that is needed to keep complications – and the surgeon – at bay.

Antacids

Antacids neutralize acid that has already been produced by the stomach. For many hiatus hernia sufferers all that is needed is an acceptable antacid that they can take whenever the symptoms arise. They can take as many as they wish, after meals and when they have heartburn. The choice of antacid is the patient's – there are many different remedies to choose from, and their pharmacist is as knowledgeable as their doctor about them.

If something a little longer-acting is needed you may be prescribed a combination of an antacid with an alginate, a medicine derived from seaweed that forms a sticky alkaline barrier against the gastric juices. This reduces reflux and helps avoid contact between the acid stomach juices and the oesophagus. Among the alginate-containing compounds (some are combined with antacid, some with H2 antagonists, for which see below) are Algitec, Gastrocote, Gastron, Gaviscon, Pyrogastrone and Topal.

A combination of antacid with a silicone (dimethylpolysiloxane, or dimethicone) may be used in similar circumstances. The silicone reduces surface tension and acts as a 'de-foaming' agent, which is thought to make it easier to belch and to allow more rapid passage of food and digestive juices through the stomach, reducing reflux as it does so. Preparations containing dimethicone include Actronorm,

Altacite Plus, Asilone, Diovol, Infacol, Kolanticon, Maalox, Simeco and Unigest.

All these preparations are popular over-the-counter drugs, which must mean that they work at least to some extent – but they have not been satisfactorily proven to do so in good, large-scale trials. All I can say here about them is that if they suit you, you may as well stick with them. However, if you are in need of them every day, you probably need to step up your medical treatment into a regimen that has been proved to work. Such a regimen usually includes drugs that suppress acid secretion by the stomach – the H2 antagonists and the proton pump inhibitors.

Acid-suppressants

Acid-suppressant drugs act by stopping the stomach from secreting acid. The first ones to be introduced were the H2 antagonists. H2 stands for histamine-2 receptor. This is part of the chemical mechanism which the stomach uses for making acid. By blocking it, these drugs greatly reduce acid production. H2 antagonists reduce rather than completely eliminate acid from the stomach – but the reduction is enough to make a very clear difference to the amount of acid refluxing through the cardia, and to be of great benefit in oesophagitis.

The H2 antagonists

Cimetidine, or Tagamet, was the first H2 antagonist. It revolutionized the treatment of gastric and peptic ulcers; it was marginally less successful in oesophagitis caused by hiatus hernia – many patients found that the symptoms, but not the oesophagitis (as assessed by endoscopy), decreased. The dose of cimetidine for hiatus hernia ranges from 400 mg four times daily to 800 mg each evening. Patients may find they have to experiment with different doses before they can settle on what is best for them.

Ranitidine (Zantac) was the second H2 antagonist. It is very similar in effect to cimetidine in relieving symptoms, although one large report suggested that it was more effective than cimetidine in healing oesophagitis. A single 300 mg dose in the evening is now preferred (rather than 150 mg twice daily). Patients who do not heal on this dose can be given doses up to 1,500 mg daily (not a dose that is often used) to get added benefit.

Newer H2 antagonists include famotidine (Pepcid) and nizatidine (Axid, Zinga); they seem to be similar to ranitidine and cimetidine, with no particular advantages over them.

Proton pump inhibitors

The first of the proton pump inhibitors was omeprazole (Losec). It was followed by lansoprazole (Zoton), and then by a host of others, that are distinguished from other drugs by having the suffix oprazole. Among them are esomeprazole (Nexium), pantoprazole (Protium) and rabeprazole (Pariet). It is doubtful whether any of these drugs has a particular advantage over any other, but doctors often prefer one of them over the others based on their own experience of its effects and side-effects. Proton pump inhibitors are much more powerful blockers of stomach secretions than H2 antagonists, so one dose can completely remove all acid from the stomach, and therefore from an irritated oesophagus, for a full 24 hours. They improve symptoms and heal oesophagitis faster than ranitidine or cimetidine.

Separate studies have shown that patients failing to respond to cimetidine or to ranitidine improved on omeprazole. In fact, all the patients who failed to heal on ranitidine healed on omeprazole. The trials suggest that 90 per cent of patients with oesophagitis heal on omeprazole treatment, either with one dose of 20 mg or 40 mg daily, given for four to 12 weeks. Lansoprazole is probably as effective as omeprazole, but the clinical evidence for its action is not as comprehensive; omeprazole remains the leading drug in this field.

Given these results, it may be surprising that everyone with oesophagitis is not given omeprazole – and I sympathize with this view. However, in these days of cost-consciousness about medical treatment, if everyone with heartburn were given omeprazole, it would greatly increase the immediate costs of health-care, possibly to the detriment of other needy groups of patients. Omeprazole still tends, therefore, to be reserved for people who have failed to heal on less expensive treatment (such as careful lifestyle management plus an antacid or an H2 antagonist), or whose severe symptoms obviously need urgent treatment.

Antacids and acid suppressants are not the only choices for people with hiatus hernias and acid reflux: other groups of drugs include the motility enhancers and the mucosal protectors.

Motility enhancers

Motility enhancers (or prokinetics) aim to increase the pressure of the sphincter between the oesophagus and the stomach, and to promote normal peristalsis. They include bethanechol (Myotonine), cisapride (Alimix, Prepulsid), domperidone (Motilium) and meto-clopramide (Gastrobid, Gastromax, Maxolon).

Of these drugs, cisapride appears to have been proved the best, in that trials have shown it to be better than metoclopramide in reducing symptoms and improving oesophagitis, to have fewer side-effects than the other motility enhancers, and to be as effective as ranitidine and cimetidine for treating oesophagitis. Added to cimetidine, it improved its effect. Its main drawback is that it causes diarrhoea and cramps in the abdomen in 5 per cent of people taking it.

Mucosal protectors

Three drugs – carbenoxolone (Bioplex, Pyrogastrone), sucralfate (Antepsin) and tripotassium dicitratobismuthate (De-Nol) – are known as mucosal protective agents. They are probably more useful against stomach and duodenal ulcers than against oesophagitis, because they are present in the lower oesophagus for too little time to make much difference. They have no effect on acid production or on gut motility; they appear to alter the quality of the mucus in the stomach and oesophagus so that it protects the underlying lining cells against acid and pepsin attack.

Studies have shown that Pyrogastrone (actually a combination of carbenoxolone and an alginate) healed oesophageal ulcers more effectively than an antacid alone, and that it was as effective as cimetidine in reducing symptoms and healing oesophagitis.

A drawback to carbenoxolone is that it can cause retention of salt and water, so it can raise the blood-pressure of susceptible persons: care must be taken to check the blood-pressure regularly in people taking the drug for long periods.

Trials of sucralfate have had differing results: one trial showed it to be no better than a placebo (a dummy tablet) at healing reflux induced oesophagitis. Others had better success: some showed it to be as effective as an antacid-alginate combination in reducing symptoms and healing oesophagitis; while others showed it to be only slightly less effective than ranitidine or cimetidine. One study found that it helped cases of oesophagitis which had failed to respond to cimetidine or ranitidine.

A problem with sucralfate is that it must be given at least two hours before or after other frequently prescribed drugs, such as the antibiotic tetracycline, the anti-epilepsy drug phenytoin, the heart-rate regulator digoxin, and cimetidine. This is because it can interfere with their absorption or metabolism – and therefore possibly alter their effectiveness. People prescribed sucralfate must therefore know exactly how often they must take their drugs and when.

De-Nol is mainly used for gastric and duodenal ulcers, but it is also gaining a reputation for healing oesophagitis, although there are no satisfactory and comprehensive trials of it in this area. It is more often used nowadays as part of a package of two or three drugs to eradicate the bacterium Helicobacter pylori from the stomach of people with ulcers.

Eradicating Helicobacter

Helicobacter pylori is a bacterium which was first brought to the world's attention in 1982 by Dr B. J. Marshall, a young hospital physician in Perth, Western Australia. He cultured it from a specimen taken from the stomach of an ulcer patient. The story of how this turned into the scientific detective story of the twentieth century is told in detail in my book Coping with Stomach Ulcers (also published by Sheldon Press). Suffice it to say here that we now know that many stomach and duodenal ulcers are caused by infection with Helicobacter pylori, and that regimens combining various drugs have been devised to eradicate them. In this way, the ulcers have been cured, and have not recurred – as ulcers do when they heal with H2 antagonists.

On the assumption that Helicobacter pylori may also have something to do with reflux-associated oesophageal ulcers – and particularly in the oesophageal ulcers that occur in Barrett's oesophagus – some doctors are using anti-Helicobacter regimens to treat people with moderate and severe reflux oesophagitis.The jury is still out on the part played by Helicobacter in oesophageal ulcers, but anti-Helicobacter treatment seems to help some patients who are resistant to the mainstream drugs. We have to wait for published trial evidence to be sure, one way or the other.

In the meantime, two main anti-Helicobacter treatment regimens have been established. One is triple therapy, combining omeprazole or lansoprazole with a week's course of two of the three antibiotics clarithromycin, amoxycillin and metronidazole; alternatively De-Nol is combined with tetracycline and metronidazole. The other is a dual combination of ranitidine bismuth citrate (Pylorid) with either amoxycillin or clarithromycin. They are highly effective against peptic ulcers in the stomach and duodenum; whether they are as effective against oesophagitis remains to be seen.

Anticholinergics

Something must be written here about another group of drugs, the anticholinergics. They include dicyclomine (Merbentyl), pirenzepine (Gastrozepin) and propantheline (Pro-Banthine). They were much used in the past because they tended to reduce acid secretion, but at the same time they also slowed down the progress of food through the gut – not an action needed for people with oesophagitis! They also have a host of uncomfortable side-effects, such as blurred vision, constipation, and, in men with enlarged prostate glands, retention of urine. They are therefore no longer the first choice for any form of acid-ulcer disease, including oesophagitis.

Combining drug treatments

Many doctors use the belt-and-braces principle in treating more severe hiatus hernia symptoms, in that they prescribe combinations of drugs, rather than single ones. I have great sympathy with their viewpoint, and have often done so myself. However, there is little published evidence that combinations are more effective than, say, omeprazole alone, in hiatus hernia with oesophagitis.

Combination studies which have been published cover cimetidine used with alginate, with metoclopramide and with cispride. On the whole they had mixed results, and for scientific proof of benefit, more studies are needed. However, it is difficult to see how they can be done now that we have moved on to using omeprazole. General practitioners like myself are likely to use a choice of different regimens, tailored to suit each individual patient. This may mean ringing the changes between H2 antagonists and proton pump inhibitors, and adding other drugs where it seems necessary, or more convenient for, or acceptable to, the patient.

Most doctors will approach the patient with hiatus hernia and the symptoms of oesophagitis in roughly the following way:

1 Advice on general health measures, as described in Chapter 6, plus antacid tablets for the occasional bout of heartburn. If that does not work then:
2 Add an H2 antagonist to the antacid regimen, and take this combination for four to six weeks. If that does not work then:
3 Give omeprazole for up to eight weeks, then review again. This will cure more than 90 per cent of cases of oesophagitis. If that does not work, then refer for further investigation and specialist management.
4 Combinations of omeprazole or an H2 antagonist with motility promoters or mucosal protectors may be tried if there is evidence, say, of motility disorders (such as feelings of fullness and belching), or of painful swallowing (when sucralfate seems particularly effective). Where it remains difficult to control symptoms, and surgeons have recommended medical treatment only, then other combinations may be tried, empirically, rather than because there is any good evidence for them.

The reasons for referring patients for surgery, and what is done during an operation, are described in the next chapter, but before that, mention must be made of drugs that may make oesophagitis worse and must be avoided or taken with extreme care by people with hiatus hernia.

Drugs and foods to be avoided (or used with care)

Some drugs (and even some foods) actually tend to relax the sphincter between the oesophagus and the stomach, so making reflux easier. They include fats, so fatty meals should be avoided. Other foodstuffs and social habits which can promote reflux in this way include coffee, chocolate, peppermint, alcohol and tobacco. The drugs which do so include (at least under experimental conditions) theophylline, used in asthma to relieve wheeze, nitrates (such as nitroglycerine and isosorbide), given to relax the coronary arteries in angina; and the progestogens used as part of the hormone cycle in the contraceptive pill. As mentioned above, anticholinergic drugs, often given for peptic ulcers, also tend to lead to reflux.

Other drugs which may delay the emptying of the stomach into the duodenum – and which may thus create the conditions for reflux – include bronchodilator (airways-opening) drugs like salbutamol for asthma, and some calcium antagonist drugs used to lower high blood-pressure. However, their use for asthma and high blood pressure may be more important than their possible (and unproven) side-effect on oesophagitis, so they should not be stopped unless they give rise to symptoms, or make symptoms worse. This goes for all the drugs and foods mentioned above. People taking, eating or drinking them should keep their possible side-effects in mind, but not necessarily stop them unless there is good reason to do so.

9

Surgery for hiatus hernia

Taking the decision to operate on a hiatus hernia is not easy. It has been made much less difficult in recent years with the introduction of omeprazole and lansoprazole, because many more people with reflux-induced oesophagitis now respond very well to medical treatment. As failure of medical treatment has always been the main reason for surgery, this has reduced the numbers needing operations.

However, that still leaves a substantial number of sufferers from hiatus hernia for whom surgery is the only answer. Apart from the small number (less than 10 per cent) of people who do not find relief from drugs, there are some younger adults whose symptoms recur as soon as they stop their continuous medical treatment. People in this second category are often uneasy about taking drugs which completely suppress stomach acid secretion for many years. There may be some basis for this fear, in that there is a small, though only theoretical, risk of it leading to a type of tumour called gastric carcinoid. It must be stressed, however, that since omeprazole was launched in the late 1980s, and has been prescribed to many millions of people for long periods, there has been no reported rise in such tumours.

Other reasons for surgery include the appearance of complications of severe reflux, such as strictures (causing swallowing difficulties and regurgitation), or Barrett's oesophagus (with bleeding, severe pain, or the threat of perforation). Surgery is also indicated where reflux is linked to motility disorders such as achalasia or nutcracker oesophagus, and in children who have not responded to the postural therapy described in Chapter 3. Some people only develop reflux disease after a previous stomach operation for a severe peptic ulcer; they too need surgery, rather than medical treatment.

Finally, there is the small group of people (around 4 per cent of all people with a hiatus hernia) whose symptoms are not caused by reflux of acid, but by the bulk of a rolling hernia in the chest. For many of them, surgery is the only way of reducing their very distressing symptoms.

Here I must say how grateful I am to the work and the publications of Professor Alfred Cuschieri, of the University of Dundee. I am not a surgeon, so this chapter reviewing surgical treatment of hiatus hernia has necessarily had to be drawn from his huge background of knowledge and experience. In his book *Reflux Oesophagitis* (written with Drs T. P. J. Hennessy and J. R. Bennett), he admits that the ideal operation has not yet been established. There are many different operations, and each one has its share of post-operative complications.

Surgery for hiatus hernia has two main aims:

1 To return the hernia from above the diaphragm to its proper abdominal site, and to close the hiatus around the oesophagus so that this material cannot return to the chest cavity. This is the diaphragmatic repair.
2 To re-shape the junction between the stomach and the lower end of the oesophagus (the cardia) to make sure that any reflux is minimized. The usual way to do this is with fundoplication, in which part of the fundus is wrapped around the last two inches of the oesophagus, and stitched in place.

The choice of operation

Since the diaphragm lies between the chest and abdomen, it can either be approached from below, through the abdomen, or from above, through the chest. For most people with a relatively uncomplicated hiatus hernia, an abdominal operation is chosen. The choice of route, however, depends partly on your build. If your hiatus is set deeply inside the abdomen, and the angle between your lower ribs (at the lower end of the breastbone) is narrow, or if you are overweight, your surgeon may prefer to go through the chest. This is not only the easier route in such patients, but it has also proved both safer and to have a better outcome for them.

Your surgeon may also go through the chest if you have had previous abdominal surgery (perhaps on the stomach or gall-bladder), or if your oesophagus is shorter than normal (usually due to scarring from years of oesophagitis). In some people with a large rolling hernia, the surgeon may decide to open both the chest and abdomen.

Recently, laparoscopic surgery (in which the repair is done through a flexible tube, just like the endoscopy tube, which is inserted into the abdomen, leaving a minimal scar) has been developed. It is only suitable for a small group of patients with less severe reflux problems, and must be carried out by a very experienced surgeon.

This is not the place for detailed descriptions of the many different operations (often named after the surgeon who invented a particular technique). It is enough to say that the most common abdominal approach is to wrap the fundus around three-quarters of the lowest five centimetres (two inches) of the oesophagus, stitch the wrap in place, and stitch the outside surface of the wrap to the left crural muscle on the lower surface of the diaphragm. This fulfils the two purposes of creating a better one-way valve between oesophagus and stomach, and also of fixing the junction firmly in place under the diaphragm (see Figure 4 overleaf). This appears to have the fewest and least severe post-operative complications.

With the approach through the chest, the technique most preferred is called the Belsey Mark IV operation. This involves wrapping and stitching the fundus twice around the front of the lower oesophagus, and returning the hernia below the diaphragm, where the hiatus is repaired and the outer 'wrap' is stitched to the crural muscle, anchoring it there. With a smaller and tighter hiatus, and the oesophageal-stomach junction firmly fixed under the diaphragm, there is little chance of recurrence.

Many surgeons are now using a new approach to prevent reflux called endoluminal fundoplication. It avoids the need for open or laparoscopic surgery by using a flexible endoscope fitted with a camera that is passed from your mouth into your oesophagus. The surgeon can see the junction between your oesophagus and your stomach and can judge precisely where to place clips that will change the shape of the junction to prevent food or stomach acid from travelling upwards. It has two great advantages in that it avoids full anaesthesia (it is usually done under sedation so that you don't remember it) and you have a much shorter stay in hospital afterwards. Your surgeon will let you know whether it is suitable for your case.

The short oesophagus

For some people, the routine operation is not enough, because their oesophagus is too short for its lower end to be brought, without tension, into the abdomen. Short oesophagus can be a complication caused by long-standing oesophagitis, or by previous operations for hiatus hernia, or may be the result of an inherited short oesophagus from childhood.

Surgery for short oesophagus is best done in a tertiary referral centre – a hospital unit specializing in oesophageal complications. In one such operation (the Collis-Nissen operation) the oesophagus is lengthened by refashioning part of the upper stomach to turn it into a replacement lower oesophagus. In another, a length of bowel is used.

In children, surgery is delayed until after the second birthday, because more than 80 per cent of children born with a hiatus hernia respond perfectly well to medical management alone, and their hernia has disappeared by that time. The preferred operation

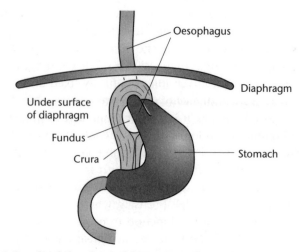

Figure 4 Result of the classical hiatus hernia repair

for most of those whose symptoms continue after their second birthday is a complete fundal wrap around the whole lower oesophagus, which is then stitched to the underside of the diaphragm. The children differ from adults in that they actually have to be tube-fed through their abdominal wall for a short time after their surgery, to allow the stomach, diaphragm and oesophagus to heal.

The results of surgery

The results of several large series of different operations to repair hiatus hernia are a tribute to the skills of modern surgeons in that the numbers of failures and problems after surgery were very small. In a report of 1,000 consecutive men and women undergoing repair of their hernias at the Emory University School of Medicine, Atlanta, Georgia, there were only 21 serious complications, and only three deaths, all in very old people with life-threatening disease. Because the surgeons used laparoscopy (in which they operate through a flexible tube, and keep cutting to a minimum), the patients, on average, were kept in hospital for only two days. Only 136 of the thousand patients had a longer hospital stay (M. Terry and colleagues, in *Surgical Endoscopy* 15(7), 2001, pp. 691–9).

Around the same time, M. L. Rogers and his colleagues in Nottingham City Hospital reported on 60 elderly patients (their average age was 69 years) who had laparoscopic surgery to repair their serious 'roller' hernias (reported in *Annals of the Royal College of Surgeons of England*, 83(6), 2001, pp. 394–8). All but one of the operations were successful: only two had heartburn afterwards, and it was controlled by proton pump inhibitors in each case.

In an even older group with rolling hernias that caused severe symptoms, with an average age of 78 years, this 'minimally invasive' laparoscopic surgery was used (K. W. Kercher and colleagues, of Charlotte, North Carolina, in *American Journal of Surgery* 182(5), 2001, pp. 510–14). It took the surgeons an average of only 61 minutes to complete the operations, and their average hospital stay afterwards was under three days. All 11 people have resumed normal eating and gained weight happily.

Sometimes the hole in the diaphragm is so large that the surgeons have to bridge the gap with a mesh, usually made of a type of polypropylene. Series of such operations have also been published, with excellent results, with no recurrence of heartburn or other symptoms (T. T. Hui and colleagues, of Los Angeles, in *American Surgeon* 67(12), 2001, pp. 1170–4).

I include these reports to reassure you that surgery for hiatus hernia is now less daunting than it may seem. You need only stay a few days at most in hospital, and you have every chance of a fast and complete recovery. If you are offered it, do consider it carefully, because the vast majority of people who accept an operation are astonished by the big improvement in the quality of life that it brings.

Strictures and bougies

A major complication of long-standing oesophagitis is stricture – a rigid narrowing of the lower oesophagus due to fibrous scarring. Strictures cause difficulties in swallowing when the inside diameter of the oesophagus shrinks to below 12 mm (around half an inch). At this level, such strictures can be relatively easily treated with medical treatment and 'bouginage'. A stricture less than three millimetres in diameter, and more than three centimetres long, proves that there is serious oesophageal disease that will probably need more extensive surgery. The higher up the oesophagus a stricture is found, the more likely it is to be due to a Barrett's oesophagus, with all the extra risks that this diagnosis entails.

The main symptom of a stricture is difficulty in swallowing: at first it is an occasional embarrassment, later (it may be months or even years in adults – it progresses faster in children) it becomes more constant. It is eventually linked with loss of weight, and sometimes bleeding and anaemia. Regurgitation from food stuck above the stricture can lead to chest infections.

After X-rays and endoscopy have established the diagnosis, the usual initial treatment is to try to open up the stricture by bouginage. This involves passing metal, spindle-shaped bougies (solid structures not unlike tiny torpedoes) over a guidewire inserted down through the stricture by means of an endoscope. The procedure starts with a small bougie, which is replaced by larger and larger bougies until the stricture is stretched to an adequate diameter.

This operation sounds horrific, but you are well prepared beforehand with an injection of a tranquillizer into a vein, and a local anaesthetic in the throat. Very nervous patients are offered a general anaesthetic, although this is rarely needed. People can usually swallow normally if their stricture diameter is increased to 15 mm. If a stricture is very rigid and resists dilation, a second session may be needed some days later.

Some people need a series of dilations before their swallowing is satisfactory, and those who still have trouble after three months of repeat dilations probably need surgery, providing they are generally fit for it.

Just removing the stricture does not remove the cause of the stricture, which is usually oesophagitis due to acid reflux – so constant medical treatment for such oesophagitis is mandatory to prevent recurrence. In the last resort, the only way to prevent recurrence may be surgical repair of the hiatus hernia and the reflux, as described in the previous few pages.

10

What's new in 2014

Asked in 2014 to update this book, I have added Martha's case (p. 12) to Chapter 1, and endoluminal fundoplication to the choices of operation (p. 87). They are small additions but significant. I have to admit that I hadn't seen a case of gastric volvulus in my many years as a GP, and may well not have recognized it if I had been her doctor. So it is a warning for anyone who is getting on in years to see your doctor quickly if you notice anything wrong in your ability to swallow or to be sick. Martha's delay of three weeks might have led to a different outcome from her current very happy one.

Endoluminal fundoplication is a welcome addition to the options for surgery in the last few years. It is now widespread and is often the first and natural choice, over open surgery and laparoscopy, for many surgeons and their patients. However, it has to be the surgeon's decision after careful consideration of the complexity of each case. So be sure, if you are faced with the choice of surgery, that you are comfortable with the choice that you and your surgeon make together on how your hernia can be cured.

I have, too, to update our knowledge on Barrett's oesophagus (pp. 28–30). In 2010, Dr Rebecca C. Fitzgerald, Medical Research Council programme leader and honorary consultant gastroenterologist at the Hutchison/MRC Research Centre, Cambridge, led a team that published the results of the use of a new screening test for Barrett's oesophagus that could be used by GPs, bypassing the need for endoscopy (Sudarshan R. Kadri and colleagues, 'Acceptability and accuracy of a non-endoscopic screening test for Barrett's oesophagus in primary care: cohort study', in *British Medical Journal* 341, 2010, c4372).

The test involves the subject swallowing, with water, a gelatine capsule containing a compressed mesh attached to a string. The string is long enough for the capsule to reach the stomach, where it lies for 5 minutes, the subject holding on to the end of the string during that time. The gelatine cover dissolves away in the stomach, leaving the mesh, now expanded, to be pulled up again. A local anaesthetic spray on the back of the throat before retrieving the mesh makes the process simple and ensures it involves minimal discomfort – far less intrusive, for example, than the usual test that involves pushing an endoscopic tube down the throat. The mesh, now retrieved, has picked up cells from the oesophagus that are identified on microscopic examination at the regional laboratory centre.

Twelve primary care practices were involved in their study, and they gathered 504 patients. Only three of them were unable to swallow the capsules, and only two of the meshes failed to expand, giving a low yield of cells. No one had any serious problems: there was no bleeding, nor was anyone sick. Barrett's oesophagus was diagnosed from testing from the type of cells recovered and from a chemical 'marker' of premalignant changes in oesophageal cells called trefoil factor 3.

The test was accurate in diagnosing Barrett's oesophagus and was well accepted by the trial patients. We are still waiting (in 2014) for larger studies to be reported, but there are encouraging signs that we might have a much more acceptable screening test for Barrett's oesophagus than the standard endoscopy that is currently used, with its much greater discomfort and cost.

Why do we need it? In the first ten years of this century we have witnessed a huge increase in cancer of the oesophagus. It is now clear that it is strongly linked to long-standing hiatus hernia with acid reflux into the oesophagus. In 2009, N. J. Shaheen and J. E. Richter reported that the incidence of oesophageal cancer, for which Barrett's oesophagus is the main risk factor, has increased six-fold in the Western world since the 1990s (N. J. Shaheen and J. E. Richter, 'Barrett's oesophagus', *The Lancet* 373, 2009, pp. 850–61). This is a huge increase – bigger than any other form of cancer.

F. Yousef and colleagues showed in 2008 that the risk of conversion from Barrett's oesophagus to cancer is 0.5 per cent per year and that the time of conversion is up to 15 years after the diagnosis is made (F. Yousef and colleagues, 'The incidence of oesophageal cancer and high-grade dysplasia in Barrett's oesophagus: a systematic review and meta-analysis', *American Journal of Epidemiology* 168, 2008, pp. 237–49).

These figures are important because if we wait until the diagnosis of cancer is made, it has an 80 per cent mortality rate in 5 years. If the condition can be identified at the Barrett's stage before cancer is diagnosed it can be treated very successfully, first by dealing with any hiatus hernia that might be allowing escape of stomach acid up into the oesophagus, and at the same time prescribing drugs like omeprazole that remove any acid from the stomach. Early cancers confined still to the lining of the oesophagus (called intraepithelial neoplasia) linked to Barrett's oesophagus are now treated in outpatient clinics using endoscopic techniques such as removal of the superficial mucus layer and 'ablating' the affected patches with radiofrequency waves.

You will gather from this that dealing with Barrett's oesophagus has become much more important, and much more effective, than it was only a decade ago – a change that was accelerated by the steep increase in oesophageal cancers and the desire to prevent them.

So my final message is that, if you have a hiatus hernia, you must take it seriously and accept that you may have to undergo unpleasant procedures to ensure that its complications (such as Barrett's oesophagus) are found early and dealt with appropriately. That course of action may well save your life.

Postscript

Perhaps the last words on hiatus hernia and oesophagitis should be left to a real expert in the disease, Professor Alfred Cuschieri. In the preface to his book, *Reflux Oesophagitis,* which is for medical readers interested professionally in the subject, he wrote that the outcome of recent research efforts had been a better appreciation of the nature of oesophagitis, and more effective drugs for its control; and that the complex relationships between reflux disease, motility disorders, abnormal circulation in the gut and chest-pain are now being unravelled. There is a growing realization, he added, that specialist treatment of the complications of oesophageal reflux disease is necessary if they are to decline, and patients are to benefit.

Professor Cuschieri's book – and his other publications on reflux disease and hiatus hernia – provide the solid framework upon which general practitioners like myself, faced daily with patients with the symptoms of hiatus hernia and oesophagitis, base our treatments. I hope that this book gives some idea of the modern expert's approach to managing a hiatus hernia without losing too many readers in technicalities.

My aim was neither to frighten readers about, nor to gloss over, the problems produced by a hiatus hernia, but to inform sufferers and their families about its modern management. It was also to translate into layman's language the knowledge I have gained in practice from treating patients and from reading the work of people like Professor Cuschieri, and his academic and surgical colleagues. In these days of the need to inform our patients about their disorders, their treatments and their likely outcome, it seems such books are needed. I hope this one has achieved its aims. Thank you for reading it!

Glossary of medical terms

achalasia   spasm of the oesophagus, leading to difficulties in swallowing

acid suppressants   drugs that stop the stomach producing acid

alginate   seaweed-derived material that forms a foam which protects the oesophagus from acid-attack

anaemia   a deficiency of red blood-cells, leading to poor oxygen supply to the body

antacids   drugs that neutralize acids formed by the stomach

antispasmodic drugs   drugs that prevent muscle-spasm and slow down peristalsis

back-flow   a condition in which material inside the gut passes upwards towards the mouth, rather than downwards, away from the mouth

bacterium   a germ that may cause infection (such as Helicobacter)

barium-swallow   an X-ray technique to show how the oesophagus and diaphragm are working

bile   the green, bitter juice produced by the liver and concentrated in the gall-bladder

biopsy   the taking of a piece of tissue for examination

bougie   an instrument designed to pass through and open up (dilate) a stricture, or narrowing, in the oesophagus

cardia   the junction between the oesophagus and the stomach

catheter   a fine, hollow tube usually used to drain fluids from the stomach

crura   the arrangement of crossed muscles that helps to hold the lower oesophagus in place under the diaphragm

crural muscle   the muscle within the crura

diaphragm   the broad sheet of muscle that separates the chest from the abdomen

diffuse spasm   a spasm that spreads all along the length of the oesophagus

dilation   widening or opening up a tube such as the oesophagus

duodenum   the first part of the small bowel, just after the stomach

dysphagia   difficulty in swallowing

endoscopy   the act of looking into an organ with a flexible fibre-optic tube

fundus   the top 10 per cent of the stomach, which lies above the cardia

gastric juices   the acid and pepsin juices produced by the stomach to start digestion

gastritis   inflammation of the stomach

gastroenterology   the study of the digestive system

haemorrhage   severe bleeding

hernia   the projection of a piece of gut into a space outside the abdomen

hernial sac   the 'bag' of membrane in which a hernia lies

herniation   the moment at which a hernia occurs

hiatus   the hole in the diaphragm through which the lower oesophagus passes

laparoscopic tube   a flexible endoscope through which surgeons operate inside the abdomen; it is passed through the abdominal wall

larynx   the voice-box, situated at the junction between the pharynx and the oesophagus

manometry   the measurement of pressure inside a hollow tube

melaena   the passing of black blood in the stools

motility   the normal movement of the muscles in the walls of the oesophagus, stomach and the rest of the gut

nutcracker oesophagus   a painful condition in which the person is aware of strong oesophageal muscle-contractions inside the chest

oblique muscles   muscles which run at an angle in the gut wall, rather than along it or around it. They keep the angle between oesophagus and stomach precisely correct

oesophagitis   inflammation of the oesophagus

oesophagus   the gullet, taking food from the throat to the stomach; it lies mainly in the chest

para-oesophageal hernia   a hernia (usually of the fundus) which comes through the diaphragm alongside the oesophagus

pepsin   a juice produced by the stomach to start to digest proteins

perforation   a hole through the wall of the oesophagus or stomach caused by an ulcer

peristalsis   the normal wave of muscle-contraction which pushes food onwards during digestion; normal peristalsis gives normal motility

pharynx   the back of the throat, between mouth and larynx

placebo   a dummy tablet with no effect, used as a comparison with new treatments to assess their effects

postural therapy   treatment for healing the oesophagus by keeping the patient upright or in a particular body position

reflux   back-flow of stomach contents upwards into the oesophagus

regimen   the overall treatment advised for a patient

regurgitation   the bringing of food which has been swallowed back into the mouth

spasm   a form of cramp in the muscles of the oesophagus

sphincter   a ring of muscle around particular areas of the gut (the cardia, the stomach–duodenum junction, the small bowel–large bowel junction and the anus), which when active stops food from passing backwards and impels it onwards

stricture   a ring-like piece of scar tissue which narrows the gut and can lead to complete blockage if not relieved

tertiary contractions   a form of peristalsis which seems to be used to churn food up, rather than pass it on; tertiary contractions cannot be felt

ulcer   a raw, punched-out area in the lining of the oesophagus, stomach or duodenum caused by the acid and/or pepsin, and the loss of the natural protection against them

waterbrash   a sour or bitter watery fluid that appears without warning in the mouth; a sign of regurgitation from the stomach

Index